List of titles

Already published

Cell Differentiation	J. M. Ashworth
Biochemical Genetics	R. A. Woods
Functions of Biological Membranes	M. Davies
Cellular Development	D. Garrod
Brain Biochemistry	H. S. Bachelard
Immunochemistry	M. W. Steward
The Selectivity of Drugs	A. Albert
Biomechanics	R. McN. Alexander
Molecular Virology	T. H. Pennington, D. A. Ritchie
Hormone Action	A. Malkinson
Cellular Recognition	M. F. Greaves
Cytogenetics of Man and other Animals	A. McDermott
RNA Biosynthesis	R. H. Burdon
Protein Biosynthesis	A. E. Smith
Biological Energy Conservation	C. Jones
Control of Enzyme Activity	P. Cohen
Metabolic Regulation	R. Denton, C. I. Pogson
Plant Cytogenetics	D. M. Moore
Population Genetics	L. M. Cook
Membrane Biogenesis	J. Haslam
Insect Biochemistry	H. H. Rees
A Biochemical Approach to Nutrition	R. A. Freedland, S. Briggs

In preparation

The Cell Cycle	S. Shall
Polysaccharides	D. A. Rees
Microbial Metabolism	H. Dalton
Bacterial Taxonomy	D. Jones
Molecular Evolution	W. Fitch
Metal Ions in Biology	P. M. Harrison, R. Hoare
Cellular Immunology	D. Katz
Muscle	R. M. Simmons
Xenobiotics	D. V. Parke
Human Genetics	J. H. Edwards
Biochemical Systematics	J. H. Harborne
Biochemical Pharmacology	B. A. Callingham
Biological Oscillations	A. Robertson

OUTLINE STUDIES IN BIOLOGY

Editor's Foreword

The student of biological science in his final years as an undergraduate and his first years as a graduate is expected to gain some familiarity with current research at the frontiers of his discipline. New research work is published in a perplexing diversity of publications and is inevitably concerned with the minutiae of the subject. The sheer number of research journals and papers also causes confusion and difficulties of assimilation. Review articles usually presuppose a background knowledge of the field and are inevitably rather restricted in scope. There is thus a need for short but authoritative introductions to those areas of modern biological research which are either not dealt with in standard introductory textbooks or are not dealt with in sufficient detail to enable the student to go on from them to read scholarly reviews with profit. This series of books is designed to satisfy this need. The authors have been asked to produce a brief outline of their subject assuming that their readers will have read and remembered much of a standard introductory textbook of biology. This outline then sets out to provide by building on this basis, the conceptual framework within which modern research work is progressing and aims to give the reader an indication of the problems, both conceptual and practical, which must be overcome if progress is to be maintained. We hope that students will go on to read the more detailed reviews and articles to which reference is made with a greater insight and understanding of how they fit into the overall scheme of modern research effort and may thus be helped to choose where to make their own contribution to this effort. These books are guidebooks, not textbooks. Modern research pays scant regard for the academic divisions into which biological teaching and introductory textbooks must, to a certain extent, be divided. We have thus concentrated in this series on providing guides to those areas which fall between, or which involve, several different academic disciplines. It is here that the gap between the textbook and the research paper is widest and where the need for guidance is greatest. In so doing we hope to have extended or supplemented but not supplanted main texts, and to have given students assistance in seeing how modern biological research is progressing, while at the same time providing a foundation for self help in the achievement of successful examination results.

J.M. Ashworth, Professor of Biology, University of Essex.

Metabolic Regulation

R.M. Denton
Lecturer in Biochemistry,
University of Bristol

and

C.I. Pogson
Lecturer in Biochemistry,
University of Kent

LONDON
CHAPMAN AND HALL

A Halsted Press Book
JOHN WILEY & SONS, INC., NEW YORK

First published in 1976
by Chapman and Hall Ltd
11 New Fetter Lane, London EC4P 4EE
© *1976 R.M. Denton and C.I. Pogson*
Printed in Great Britain
at the University Printing House, Cambridge

ISBN 0 412 13150 1

Distributed in the U.S.A.
by Halsted Press, a Division
of John Wiley & Sons, Inc. New York

Library of Congress Cataloging in Publication Data

Denton, Richard Michael.
  Metabolic regulation.

  (Outline studies in biology)
  Includes bibliographies and index.
  1. Metabolic regulation. I. Pogson, C.I.,
joint author. II. Title.
QP171.D46   599'.01'33   76-13455
ISBN 0-470-15126-9

Contents

Introduction

The regulation of biochemical processes may be viewed from a number of different perspectives, ranging from that of the physiologist (specifically including those concerned with hormonal interrelationships) to that of the molecular enzymologist. To these we should also add those interested in developmental biology and differentiation where regulation is of a more permanent and long-term nature. In this book, we have concentrated on aspects which concern us most closely in our own research, namely the control and interactions of intracellular metabolic pathways.

The individual steps in most metabolic pathways have been well known for a decade or more and are well described in a number of general biochemical textbooks. The mechanisms responsible for regulation are in general not so well understood despite much research effort in recent years. One of the principal objectives of this book is to try to give the reader not only a general survey of the types of mechanism which can modulate fluxes through metabolic pathways, but also an understanding of the difficulties and complexities which can beset the researcher who seeks to establish unequivocally the mechanism responsible for initiating an observed change in flux through a metabolic pathway in a particular circumstance.

The general strategy and tactics employed in the study of metabolic regulation are covered in Chapters 1 and 2 which deal in turn with the theoretical and practical aspects of the subject. The final chapter considers in depth regulation of specific pathways. A virtually universal problem, and one which seems to be limiting progress in many areas, is the compartmentation of intermediary metabolites and enzymes in cells. Much attention has been placed in this book on the occurrence of compartmentation and the reasons why it interferes with investigations of control mechanisms.

The bias of the authors towards mammalian metabolism becomes increasingly evident in Chapters 2 and 3. A small book has to be selective, particularly in the range of examples that can be presented. We have chosen in Chapter 3 to concentrate on selected aspects of the metabolism of heart muscle, adipose tissue and liver. All are concerned with the metabolism and interrelationships of carbohydrate and fat, the major fuels. Taken as a whole, it is hoped that this chapter will give a useful outline of present knowledge of the regulation of mammalian fuel and energy metabolism, especially during the important feeding — fasting and excercise — rest cycles.

At the end of each chapter we have listed specific references together with suggestions for further reading. We are acutely aware that these lists are incomplete and, in particular, that many important original papers are omitted. We hope that the authors of these papers will forgive us — the subject, even those aspects covered in this book, has an enormous bibliography. Most of the articles cited are either of recent date or are selected review articles which in turn include references to original articles.

1 Theoretical aspects of metabolic regulation

1.1 Definitions

Before embarking on detailed discussions of the principles of metabolic regulation, the reader may find it helpful to have some guidance as to the terminology and concepts that will be subsequently assumed.

Firstly, the word 'regulatory' itself. One may study the problems of intermediary metabolism in several ways. One is to examine the behaviour of whole complex systems; another is to attempt to isolate specific enzymes and investigate their kinetic properties. Following this latter approach, researchers have been able to show that the activities of certain enzymes may be controlled *in vitro* by changes in the concentration of physiological compounds other than the immediate substrates and/or products. This control may take the form of activation or inhibition and be exerted either on the catalytic efficiency of the enzyme (i.e. V_{max} effects) or upon the tightness of binding of the substrate to the active site (i.e. K_m effects). Such behaviour is generally described as 'regulatory', and is often rationalized in terms of the role of the enzyme in question in its physiological context.

It is, of course, a truism to say that every metabolic pathway can and must have only one 'rate-limiting' step. The techniques and methods by which this step can be pinpointed will be discussed in detail below. Several pathways, however, include more than one enzyme which has been described at some time as 'regulatory'. Clearly not all can be simultaneously rate-limiting. It is nevertheless possible for the locus of the rate-limiting step to change as conditions change (e.g. variation in substrate and/or oxygen supply, availability of hormones, general nutritional conditions, etc.), so that there may be two or more enzymes with a physiological 'regulatory' function in any pathway. Not infrequently, however, the metabolic data has failed to live up to the enzymologists' expectation, to the extent that no rate-limiting role can be discerned for a particular enzyme with apparent 'regulatory' properties. As an example, we may consider L-glutamate dehydrogenase which catalyses the reaction

$$\text{L-glutamate} + \text{NAD}^+ \rightleftharpoons \text{2-oxoglutarate} + \text{NADH} + \text{NH}_4^+. \qquad (1.1)$$

The purified enzyme is activated *in vitro* by ADP and L-leucine and inhibited by very low concentrations of GTP. Because of these properties, it has been proposed at various times that the enzyme may control either the rate of glutamate synthesis from 2 oxoglutarate or vice versa. The opposing view has been that this step is at equilibrium and could therefore not be rate-limiting in either direction! Indeed, the K_{eq} for glutamate dehydrogenase has been used for calculation of the mitochondrial NADH/NAD$^+$ ratio; this in many instances gives results similar to those obtained using another mitochondrial dehydrogenase, β-hydroxybutyrate dehydrogenase [1]. Nevertheless evidence is now accruing which indicates that, under some conditions at least, the enzyme may be rate-limiting for glutamate synthesis [2]. In the same way, time may well show that the regulatory properties observed *in vitro* for other enzymes, not presently recognized as rate-limiting, may be relevant to their activities *in vivo*.

From this brief discussion, it should be clear that 'regulatory' is a term which is used far more loosely and widely than 'rate-limiting', and is one which should be subject to some scrutiny when extrapolation is made from isolated enzyme studies to more complex biological situations.

The term 'pathway' has already been used and will figure frequently in this book. From the point of view of metabolic regulation, a pathway is best defined as a sequence of intermediates between two branch points. Thus, in the sequence

$$A \rightarrow B \rightarrow C \rightarrow D \rightarrow E \rightarrow F$$
$$\downarrow \qquad\qquad\quad \downarrow$$
$$X \rightarrow Y \qquad\quad Z$$

there may be said to be five pathways: $A \rightarrow B$, $B \rightarrow E$, $E \rightarrow F$, $B \rightarrow Y$ and $E \rightarrow Z$, each with its own rate-limiting reaction. Although this is a convenient theoretical definition, in practice 'pathway' is used more widely. The 'glycolytic pathway', for example, is usually understood to include the reactions between glucose and pyruvate (or lactate). This sequence, however, includes a number of possible branch points; for example at glucose 6-phosphate, which may be converted into glycogen, back into glucose, or provide pentose phosphate as well as feeding into the glycolytic chain. Glycolytic flux from glucose therefore passes through at least two operational 'pathways', each subject to control, namely, glucose $\rightarrow$ glucose 6-phosphate and glucose 6-phosphate $\rightarrow$ triose phosphates, etc.

For the present we shall eschew pedantry and use 'pathway' in both senses, trusting that the context will avoid ambiguity. We should remind the reader nevertheless that confusion about regulatory mechanisms arising from misunderstandings about 'pathways' is by no means absent from the biochemical literature.

1.2 Identification of rate-limiting steps

In any one pathway under steady-state conditions, the rate of net substrate utilization equals the rate of net product output. It follows that the *net* rate (that is, the amount by which the 'forward' exceeds the 'back' rate) through each enzymic step is the same. Where enzymes have high activities, both 'back' and 'forward' rates will be substantially greater than the net rate and the reactions will be essentially at equilibrium; in contrast, the rate-limiting enzyme will have little or no back rate and thus a forward rate close to the net rate.

An understanding of the regulation of the pathway requires first the identification of the rate-limiting step and then the recognition of the factors responsible for changes in activity of the enzyme catalysing this step in any one circumstance. There are two definitive methods whereby a rate-limiting reaction may be clearly pinpointed (see 1.2.1 and 1.2.2) but often circumstantial evidence can be obtained by other techniques (see 1.2.3).

1.2.1 Measurement of the mass action ratio

The mass action ratio (M.A.R.) may be defined as the ratio of the concentrations of the product(s) to those of the substrate(s) under given conditions. Where a reaction is at equilibrium the M.A.R. equals K'_{eq}, the apparent equilibrium constant; if the reaction is non-equilibrium, the two values will diverge. Although there is no hard-and-fast rule, in general enzymes that are rate-limiting exhibit M.A.R.s 2–4 orders of magnitude smaller than the K'_{eq}. The discrepancy, if any, between M.A.R. and K'_{eq} for other reactions is far less, sufficiently small to be explicable on grounds of experimental error or, metabolic compartmentation, or variation in K'_{eq} with changes in pH or metal ion concentration. Examples of the calculation of M.A.R.s are given in Fig. 1.1.

1.2.2 Measurement of reaction rates

There are instances where measurements of

(a) *Pyruvate kinase*

$$\text{Phosphoenolpyruvate} + \text{ADP} \rightleftharpoons \text{Pyruvate} + \text{ATP}; K'_{eq} = 0.6 \times 10^4$$

Conc. in liver

Phosphoenolpyruvate	$7 \times 10^{-5} \, \text{M}$
Pyruvate	$3 \times 10^{-5} \, \text{M}$
ATP	$3.75 \times 10^{-3} \, \text{M}$
ADP	$1.88 \times 10^{-3} \, \text{M}$

(Data from [3]).

$$\text{M.A.R.} = \frac{[\text{Pyruvate}] \, [\text{ATP}]}{[\text{Phosphoenolpyruvate}] \, [\text{ADP}]} = \frac{(3 \times 10^{-5})(3.75 \times 10^{-3})}{(7 \times 10^{-5})(1.88 \times 10^{-3})} = 0.85$$

From comparison with K'_{eq}, the reaction is clearly far displaced from equilibrium, and pyruvate kinase is rate-limiting. The discrepancy between the two values is sufficiently great that it cannot reasonably be argued that special factors, such as compartmentation, are involved.

(b) *Nucleoside diphosphate kinase*

$$\text{ATP} + \text{GDP} \rightleftharpoons \text{ADP} + \text{GTP}; K'_{eq} \approx 1.$$

Conc. in liver

ATP	$2.36 \times 10^{-3} \, \text{M}$
ADP	$0.97 \times 10^{-3} \, \text{M}$
GTP	$0.63 \times 10^{-3} \, \text{M}$
GDP	$0.21 \times 10^{-3} \, \text{M}$

(Data from [4]).

$$\text{M.A.R.} = \frac{[\text{ADP}] \, [\text{GTP}]}{[\text{ATP}] \, [\text{GDP}]} = \frac{(0.97 \times 10^{-3})(0.63 \times 10^{-3})}{(2.36 \times 10^{-3})(0.21 \times 10^{-3})} = 1.23$$

Since the M.A.R. and K'_{eq} values are so close to each other, one may safely say that the enzyme is in equilibrium *in vivo*.

Fig. 1.1 Comparison of mass action ratios and equilibrium constants.

metabolites are impracticable or difficult to interpret (e.g. because of compartmentation effects, see 1.3.2). In these cases it may be possible to measure the forward and backward rates more directly using isotopically-labelled substrates.

If we consider the sequence:

$$A \rightarrow B \rightarrow C \rightarrow D \rightarrow E \rightarrow \dots.$$

and imagine that, for example, ^{14}C-labelled A is added, then each of the compounds B to E etc. will be labelled in turn with [14]C. If the rate of the reaction $A \rightarrow B$ is rapid in comparison with the net flux along the pathway, the ^{14}C specific activity of B will rise rapidly to that of A. Similar arguments apply to all reactions other than that which is not in equilibrium (i.e. the rate-limiting step). In this case the rate of the 'back' reaction will be near zero and the product will be relatively slow in reaching isotopic equilibrium with the corresponding substrate. In practice, therefore, a study of the changes in specific activity of metabolic intermediates as a function of time will identify the controlling steps in the pathway. An example of this technique is described in Section 3.2.3.

1.2.3 Circumstantial evidence

(i) *Theoretical grounds.* From a teleological standpoint, it is advantageous to avoid undue accumulation of intermediates in a pathway, since such accumulation is energetically wasteful. One may therefore initially expect that rate-limiting steps will be found at, or close to, the start of any metabolic sequence [5]. From previous experience, one might look first at those enzymes catalysing reactions involving large free energy changes. However, although many non-equilibrium reactions do exhibit large and negative $\Delta G^{0\prime}$ values (e.g. phosphofructokinase, $\Delta G^{0\prime} = -17.6$ kJ/mol; pyruvate dehydrogenase, $\Delta G^{0\prime} = -39.4$ kJ/mol), there is no *necessary* correlation between these two characteristics. Thus, lactate dehydrogenase catalyses a step probably always at equilibrium with $K'_{eq} = 9 \times 10^3$ (in the direction of pyruvate reduction; $\Delta G^{0\prime} = -23.5$ kJ/mol) whilst glycogen phosphorylase and glucose transport in certain tissues are rate-limiting steps with K_{eq} values equal or near to unity. Thus, theory may give merely a rough indication of those enzymes whose investigation might yield dividends.

(ii) *Addition of intermediates.* If, in a sequence — $A \rightarrow B \rightarrow C \rightarrow D \rightarrow E \rightarrow F$ the reaction $B \rightarrow C$ is limiting, then addition of C, D or E will lead to an increase in the rate of appearance of F. Since added A or B have to pass the 'bottleneck' at $B \rightarrow C$, rates with these precursors will be similar to those in the control situation. By suitable addition of intermediates, therefore, it should be possible to locate the rate-limiting step. Two problems frequently (indeed, usually) arise — (a) intermediates may fail to stimulate not because they are 'before' the rate-limiting step, but because they are transported to the system (i.e. across membrane barriers) poorly or not at all; and, (b) the concentrations added may be such that the regulatory properties of the system are altered.

(iii) *Properties of enzymes.* A rough indication of regulatory enzymes may be obtained from measurements of maximum activities *in vitro.* It is reasonable to expect that those enzymes which are present in amounts in excess ($10^2 - 10^4$ fold) of those required for maintenance of the overall rates are not regulatory. Conversely, enzymes whose activity is only a little greater than that minimally required may well be regulators. Once again, difficulties in interpretation are frequently encountered. Firstly, some enzymes known to be regulatory do occur at moderately excessive concentrations; only a small proportion of their total activity is expressed *in vivo* (e.g. liver pyruvate kinase). Secondly, there are examples of non-regulatory enzymes whose activity is relatively low — aldolase is an example [6].

In addition, there are practical difficulties. Enzymes are usually assayed *in vitro* at great dilution and in media far removed from the physiological condition (see Chapter 2). Thus maximum activities in the laboratory may be only a rough guide. Some progress has been made towards assaying enzymes *in vivo*, either with highly specific isotopic methods [7] or by artificially increasing membrane permeability to substrates [8]. Problems may also arise where an enzyme exists in interconvertible forms; unless the physiological ratio of the various forms is preserved during extraction and *in vitro,* large errors in V_{max} determination may occur.

Further information may be obtained by more detailed kinetic analysis of enzymes suspected of regulatory function. The occurrence of co-operative and allosteric behaviour, particularly if such properties make sense physiologically, is powerful, albeit not conclusive (see 1.1), evidence that an enzyme may be important in metabolic control.

In micro-organisms, in particular, there is generally much more information about the properties of potentially regulatory enzymes *in vitro* and the total metabolic flux through them *in vivo*, than there is about the concentra-

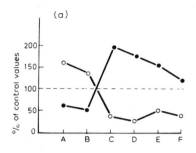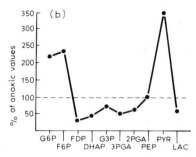

Fig. 1.2 Cross-over plots. (a) Diagrammatic. When the flow A → F increases (●—●), [B] decreases, suggesting that B → C may be the rate-limiting step. Conversely, when flow decreases (o—o), [B] rises. (b) Plot of glycolytic intermediates in the perfused rat heart during recovery from anoxia. The control condition is anoxic perfusion; the values after 5 min of aerobic perfusion (when glycolytic flux is depressed) are expressed as percentages of those in anoxia. From this and other experiments, it is clear that phosphofructokinase is here the rate-limiting enzyme; the cross-over at lactate dehydrogenase is due to changes in the NADH/NAD$^+$ ratio. G6P – glucose 6-phosphate; F6P – fructose 6-phosphate; FDP – fructose 1,6-diphosphate; DHAP – dihydroxyacetone phosphate; G3P – glyceraldehyde 3-phosphate; 3PGA – 3-phosphoglycerate; 2PGA – 2-phosphoglycerate; PEP – phosphoenolpyruvate; PYR – pyruvate; LAC – lactate. From [11].

tions of the substrates and products of the relevant pathways. There is thus a dearth of *direct* evidence for the rate-limiting role of any particular enzyme, and we are at present largely dependent on the type of indirect, circumstantial, evidence described above and on experiments involving mutant organisms with specific alterations or deletions of enzymes in the pathway under scrutiny.

(iv) *Cross-over plots.* In the course of the investigation into the sequence of carriers in the mitochondrial electron transport chain, Chance and Williams [9] noted that, during ADP limitation, components close to oxygen became more oxidized, whilst those nearer the substrate end of the chain were correspondingly more reduced. Similar experiments with site-specific inhibitors led Chance and his colleagues [9,10] to develop the *cross-over theorem.* This may best be explained if we look again at a theoretical pathway

$$A \overset{a}{\rightleftharpoons} B \overset{b}{\rightarrow} C \overset{c}{\rightleftharpoons} D \overset{d}{\rightarrow} E \overset{e}{\rightarrow} F.$$

If the rate of carbon flow from A to F is in-

creased (by direct activation or removal of inhibitor), then the flow through the rate-limiting step (for the sake of example, at enzyme b) must, by definition, be increased equally. Under the original conditions, the limiting activity of b results in an accumulation of the equilibrium mixture of A and B. Correspondingly, the relatively higher activities of enzymes c, d and e contribute to a low steady-state level of C. When the activity of b increases relative to the activities of the other four enzymes, then the concentrations of A and B will fall, and that of C may rise, until new steady-state values are attained. In a cross-over plot (Fig. 1.2) the ratio new steady-state concentration/control steady-state concentration expressed as a percentage of the control is plotted against the metabolic sequence. Cross-overs are obtained when the lines joining the % ratios of substrate and product cross the 100% line. When such cross-overs result from *either* increased substrate concentration where total flow is decreased or vice versa, then they may indicate rate-limiting sites. One cannot, however, draw any firm conclusions where the cross-over is produced in other ways. Equally, the absence of a cross-over does not mean that a particular enzyme is not regulatory. For example, a non-equilibrium reaction controlled by substrate availability alone, such as pyruvate kinase in heart muscle, will not be revealed by such a plot.

Cross-over plots involve many assays (not always feasible), are time consuming, and may not be possible where the pathway is very short. It is clear that the conclusions to be drawn are solely dependent on the contrary changes in substrate concentration and metabolic flux, so that measurements of these parameters alone may suffice for a given enzyme.

Most enzymes differ from the components of the electron transport chain studied in Chance's laboratory, in that they act upon more than one substrate and produce more than one product. Since the other components involved are frequently nucleotides (e.g. $NAD^+/NADH$ or ATP/ADP) whose concentration ratios may be greatly affected by extraneous factors, it follows that misinterpretation of cross-overs can readily occur; it is possible to get an apparent cross-over at a step catalysed by a dehydrogenase or a kinase which is near equilibrium.

Without doubt, the safer strategy is to attempt first to obtain evidence that the step concerned is out of equilibrium, and then to compare changes in substrate concentration with changes in flux. Parallel changes in substrate concentration and flux suggest that the change in flux is initiated by the change in substrate concentration. Inverse changes in substrate concentration and flux indicate that the change in flux derives from a change in the activity of the enzyme catalysing this particular step. Studies would then be focussed on the mechanisms which bring about this change in enzyme activity.

1.3 Regulatory factors

1.3.1 Introduction
All enzyme-catalysed reactions may be des-

cribed by appropriate modifications of the simple reaction scheme

$$E + S \rightleftharpoons ES \rightarrow E + P.$$

The rate of reaction is a function of the concentrations of 'active' substrate, $[S]_{active}$, and of 'active' enzyme $[E]_{active}$. The $[S]_{active}$ is that proportion of the total substrate which is in the appropriate conformation for direct binding to the enzyme; the $[E]_{active}$ is conversely the proportion of enzyme molecules which may react directly with substrate. In this context, the term enzyme may be broadened to include membrane carriers ('vectorial' enzymes) and hormone receptors, whether membrane-bound or soluble.

Changes in reaction rate are effected only through changes in $[S]_{active}$, $[E]_{active}$, or both. It is important to emphasise that $[S]_{active}$ and $[E]_{active}$ are not necessarily directly related to the total concentrations of substrate or enzyme.

1.3.2 Control through $[S]_{active}$
(a) *Limitation by total substrate availability.* Most enzymes catalyse equilibrium reactions *in vivo*. Their kinetic behaviour in both forward and reverse directions is generally simple (Michaelis-Menten). The concentrations of substrates (and products) for these enzymes are often close to the K_m value.

The net rate through non-equilibrium reactions can be limited by substrate concentration. This can only occur if the substrate concentration is near or below the K_m value. In such cases, the rate through the step is being determined by the activity of another enzyme catalysing a previous step in the sequence.

(b) *Physical unavailability of substrate.* In the eukaryotic cell there are numerous distinct membrane-bound compartments, e.g. nuclei, cytoplasm, mitochondria, lysosomes, etc. Many common metabolites occur in more than one compartment of the cell. Thus, nucleoside triphosphates are involved both in transcription, which is nuclear, and in translation, which is

Table 1.1 Anionic porter systems in rat liver mitochondria. The inhibitors have been important in distinguishing and characterizing the various systems in isolated mitochondria. Not all penetrate into whole tissue, and others may have non-specific side effects, which must be checked in each experimental situation.

Anion	Counter-ion	Inhibitors
phosphate	hydroxyl	-SH reagents
malate, succinate	phosphate	butylmalonate
citrate, isocitrate	malate, (phosphoenolpyruvate)	$\Big\{$ 2-ethylcitrate benzene 1, 2, 3-tricarboxylate
2 oxoglutarate	malate	
glutamate	hydroxyl	avenaceolide
aspartate	glutamate + H^+	
pyruvate	hydroxyl	α-cyano-4-hydroxy-cinnamate
ATP	ADP	atractyloside, bongkrekic acid

cytoplasmic, as well as serving as precursors and energy sources throughout the cell. They may also be associated with tissue-specific organelles such as the adrenaline-containing granules of the adrenal medulla [12] and the nucleotide storage granules in the eggs of the brine shrimp, *Artemia salina* [13]. It is not unreasonable, therefore, to expect that nucleotides may not be evenly distributed throughout the cell, and that they may be present at different concentrations in the several organelles involved. There is indeed strong evidence that physical compartmentation is a real and important phenomenon in eukaryotes. Even in prokaryotes, where the general absence of membrane-bound organelles makes it more difficult to envisage simple compartmentation, there is strong isotopic evidence for different 'pools' of nucleotides [14].

Little attention has been paid to metabolic 'pools' on either side of the nuclear membrane. The composition of the mitochondrial matrix is, however, known to be distinct from that of the cytoplasm. The inner mitochondrial membrane contains porter systems which selectively permit the passage of certain intermediates; in general, the membrane is impermeable to charged compounds.

The various porter systems in liver mitochondria are listed in Table 1.1. It should be noted that transport of many anionic intermediates is linked either directly (e.g. pyruvate, phosphate) or indirectly (e.g. malate, citrate) to the transport of hydroxyl groups. Distribution of these anions across the mitochondrial membrane may be determined by the pH gradient generated by respiration; in general it would be expected that the concentration of the anions within the mitochondria would be greater than that in the cytoplasm.

Mitochondria can exchange exogenous with endogenous adenine nucleotide, providing that there is a 1:1 exchange of adenine moieties across the membrane. The net effect is that the total concentrations of adenine nucleotide inside and outside the mitochondrion are constant, but that the phosphorylation state in both compartments may, in theory at least, be in equilibrium. Nucleotides such as GTP cannot cross the mitochondrial membrane, and are presumably dependent for rephosphorylation on the adenine nucleotide porter and nucleoside diphosphate kinase activity (Fig. 1.3).

Reducing equivalents may enter and leave the mitochondrion as malate:

$$\text{oxaloacetate} + \text{NADH} + \text{H}^+ \underset{\textit{malate dehydrogenase}}{\rightleftharpoons} \text{malate} + \text{NAD}^+$$

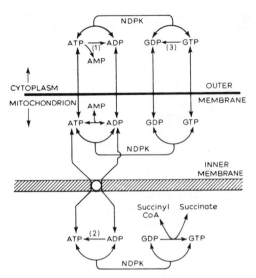

Fig. 1.3 Interrelationships between adenine and guanine nucleotide metabolism. Note that adenine nucleotides only can cross the inner mitochondrial membrane via a specific porter system. (1) Biosynthetic energy-requiring processes, (2) Electron transport, (3) Protein synthesis, microtubular and hormonal activity. NDPK – Nucleoside diphosphate kinase.

Note that the NAD moiety itself does not cross the membrane (Fig. 1.4). The complete carbon skeleton of oxaloacetate, on the other hand, can cross the membrane as malate or as aspartate (Fig. 1.4), although the membrane is virtually impermeable to oxaloacetate itself.

As well as binding to their specific enzymes, substrates may interact with other cellular components *in vivo* and, in so doing, may reduce their 'active' concentration. Aconitate hydratase catalyses the interconversion of citrate and *threo* $D_s(+)$ isocitrate. Increasing the Mg^{2+} concentration *in vitro* raises the proportion of citrate in the equilibrium mixture. This results from the tighter binding of Mg^{2+} to citrate than to isocitrate, and from the enzyme's inability to bind either metal complex. The overall reaction is therefore

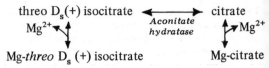

From comparison of the K'_{eq} for aconitate hydratase at various concentrations of Mg^{2+} *in vitro* with the M.A.R., one may get some estimate of the concentration of Mg^{2+} available to the enzyme *in vivo*; this is only a very small fraction of the total Mg^{2+} present [15]. Most intracellular Mg^{2+} is bound to ATP as $ATP\ Mg^{2-}$ (some is bound to ADP and proteins such as myosin and tubulin). The apparent equilibrium positions of adenylate kinase and creatine phosphokinase are also sensitive to changes in $[Mg^{2+}]$ and measurements of the M.A.R. of these reactions have also been used to estimate $[Mg^{2+}]$.

Where an enzyme is present at concentrations greater than its substrate, then that substrate may be effectively totally bound. An example is the glyceraldehyde 3-phosphate dehydrogenase (GAPDH) – 3-phosphoglycerate kinase (PGK) sequence in the glycolytic chain. The concentrations of the enzymes *in vivo* are of the order of 10^{-4} M, whilst that of 1, 3-diphosphoglycerate is below 10^{-5} M. Hess [16] has shown that there is a 1:1 correspondence of the subunits of GAPDH and PGK in yeast; this is consistent with direct transfer of 1,3-diphosphoglycerate from one enzyme to the other.

M.A.R. measurements of the triose phosphate isomerase equilibrium in mammalian tissues reveal that there is a small but consistent deviation from the expected K'_{eq} despite the high enzyme activity. This may be ascribed to the low concentrations of the triose phosphates in relation to the concentrations of the binding sites of GAPDH, triose phosphate isomerase, L-glycerol 1-phosphate dehydrogenase and aldolase. The 'active' concentrations of substrate available to triose phosphate isomerase may therefore be very much less than the total present; acid-extraction will, of course, release any

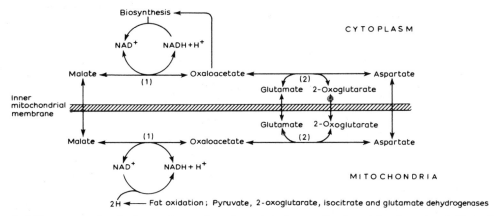

Fig. 1.4 Transport of reducing power and oxaloacetate from mitochondrion to cytosol. Note that reducing equivalents, but not NADH itself, leave the mitochondrion. Oxaloacetate leaves as malate when cytosolic NADH is limiting (through the action of distinct mitochondrial and cytoplasmic malate dehydrogenases (1) or as aspartate, involving transamination with distinct glutamate-oxaloacetate transaminases (2). The inner mitochondrial membrane only is shown; metabolites cross the outer membrane by simple diffusion. Details of mitochondrial porter systems have been omitted for clarity.

enzyme-bound substrate and subsequent assays will give a total tissue content.

(c) *Chemical unavailability of substrate.* This is a consequence of the high degree of specificity in enzymic reactions, and of the occurrence of multiple forms of substrate in solution. These may take the form of various ionic species or of other interconvertible forms.

HCO_3^- is one of the primary buffers *in vivo*; it is also a substrate for synthetic carboxylation reactions (e.g. pyruvate carboxylase, acetyl CoA carboxylase, etc.). CO_2 is not a substrate for these reactions, but is the product of physiological decarboxylations (e.g. 6-phosphogluconate dehydrogenase, phosphoenolpyruvate carboxykinase). Similar specificity occurs with mitochondrial porter systems. Since electrical neutrality must be conserved, $H_2 PO_4^-$ alone can exchange with OH^-; the concentration of this ion is dependent on both the total phosphate and on the pH. Similarly, malate and citrate must exchange as divalent anions. K_m values for

such compounds should of course be expressed in terms of the concentration of the 'active' species transported.

A different type of substrate interconversion is that of the sugars, which can exist in both anomeric ($\alpha-$ and $\beta-$) forms as well as furanose, pyranose and straight chain configurations. Enzymes exhibit specificity for both of these factors (e.g. phosphoglucomutase is specific for α-glucopyranose 6-phosphate, whereas glucose 6-phosphate dehydrogenase is specific for β-glucopyranose 6-phosphate); in tissues and whole organisms the possibility of limitation by availability of either $\alpha-$ or $\beta-$anomer is unlikely, since spontaneous interconversion through straight-chain forms is rapid and is further enhanced by a ubiquitous mutarotase activity.

Metabolites with carbonyl groups may undergo both hydration and keto-enol tautomerism. Glyceraldehyde 3-phosphate (G3P) exists at 37°C as 95.7% in the hydrated form, and only 4.3% in the aldehyde form normally shown in

15

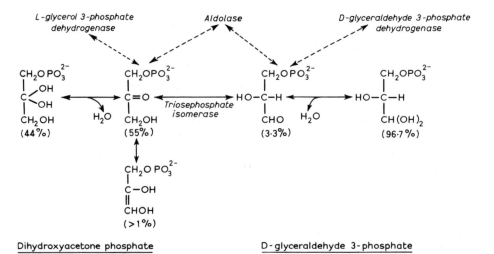

Fig. 1.5 Forms of triose phosphates. The percentages in brackets refer to the relative amounts of each triose phosphate form at equilibrium in aqueous solution at 20°C. Dotted lines indicate the forms bound by the enzymes shown.

biochemical texts (Fig. 1.5). Since the enzymes which act on glyceraldehyde 3-phosphate are all specific for the free aldehyde, their K_m values for glyceraldehyde 3-phosphate are 4.3/100 times those obtained by calculation from the total G3P concentration. Dihydroxyacetone phosphate exhibits similar behaviour, and has a small proportion of the enolic species (Fig. 1.5).

Oxaloacetate is a particularly significant compound in that it is a crucial intermediate in several major metabolic sequences. Its 'active' concentration in any one case is difficult to assess; there are 'pools' in both cytoplasm and mitochondria, the concentration is sufficiently low for binding to enzymes and other compon-ents to be important, especially within mito-chondria, and there is the possibility of four interconvertible forms. At 20°C *in vitro*, 74% is in the form of the enzymic substrate, keto-oxaloacetate, 8% is 2, 2-dihydroxysuccinate and 18% is enolic forms.

1.3.3 Control through $[E]_{active}$

(a) *Physical compartmentation.* This, of course, overlaps with substrate compartmentation, since the effect is the physical separation of enzyme from substrate. Nevertheless some systems are generally considered from the enzyme's 'view', and will be so here. An ob-vious example is associated with the lysosome, one of whose functions is the containment of lytic enzymes; the primary role of these is pre-sumably in the slow digestion of cytoplasmic constituents in autophagic vacuoles where the pH is near optimal (4 to 6) for enzyme activity. In this case the teleological importance of com-partmentation is obvious. A second example is the ribonuclease which is associated with ribo-somes yet is probably 'latent' *in vivo*. This en-zyme is a problem experimentally in studies concerned with the mechanism of protein syn-thesis, since it may be readily activated and then attack both endogenous and exogenous RNA.

16

Table 1.2 Zymogen systems in mammals: some examples.

Zymogen	'Enzyme'	Type of cleavage	Comments
Trypsinogen	Trypsin	Proteolysis by entero-kinase or trypsin	Proteases in digestion
Chymotrypsinogen	Chymotrypsin	Proteolysis by trypsin	
Procarboxypeptidase	Carboxypeptidase	Proteolysis by trypsin	
Prothrombin (factor II)	Thrombin (factor IIa)	Proteolysis by activated factors	Proteases in blood clotting
Factors VII, IX, X	Factors VIIa, IXa, Xa		
Complement factors	Activated complexes	Proteolysis by activated factors	Proteases in immune response
Angiotensinogen	Angiotensin II	Proteolysis by renin and converting enzyme	Hormone stimulating aldosterone synthesis
Proinsulin	Insulin	Proteolysis by trypsin-like activity	Hormone acting on fuel metabolism
Proparathyroid hormone	Parathyroid hormone	Proteolysis	Hormone maintaining Ca^{2+} and phosphate homeostasis

Table 1.3 Enzymatically-interconvertible systems. Nos. 1–7 are well established, No. 8 onwards, less so.

Enzyme	Source	Type of Modification	*Active Species
1. Glycogen phosphorylase	Mammalian	Phosphorylation	EP
2. Phosphorylase b kinase	Mammalian	Phosphorylation	EP
3. Glycogen synthetase	Mammalian	Phosphorylation	E
4. Triglyceride lipase	Mammalian	Phosphorylation	EP
5. Pyruvate dehydrogenase	Mammalian	Phosphorylation	E
6. Glutamine synthetase	E. coli	Adenylylation	E
7. Glutamine synthetase adenylyltransferase activator (P_{II})	E. coli	Uridylylation	†E and E-UMP
8. Pyruvate kinase	Liver	Phosphorylation	E
9. Acetyl CoA carboxylase	Liver	Phosphorylation	E?
10. Tyrosine 3-hydroxylase	Brain	Phosphorylation	EP
11. Cholesterol esterase	Adipose tissue	Phosphorylation	EP
12. RNA polymerase	E. coli	Phosphorylation	?
13. Phosphofructokinase	Liver	Phosphorylation	EP?
14. Fatty acid synthetase	Liver (pigeon)	Phosphorylation	E?

*   E represents unmodified enzyme; EP, phosphorylated form. Forms not shown may be either less active or inactive.

†   E directs adenylyltransferase to adenylylate glutamine synthetase; E-UMP, the uridylyl-enzyme, directs the adenylyltransferase to convert adenylylated glutamine synthetase to the unmodified state.

(b) *Chemical compartmentation.* As with substrates, so enzymes may exist in one or more forms of different activity within the same functional region of the cell. This diversity takes three possible forms — zymogens (or pro-enzymes), interconvertible enzymes and protein-protein complexes.

Zymogen systems differ from the other two in that they appear to be all extracellular and are uni-directional, i.e. the zymogen is cleaved to yield the active species, but cannot be reconstituted save through complete proteolysis and *de novo* synthesis. This type of mechanism is also known to be important for some hormones; typical examples are listed in Table 1.2. The inactivity of the zymogen itself may protect the intracellular protein synthetic mechanism (e.g. gut enzymes) or prevent the initiation of a potentially disastrous cascade (e.g. clotting and complement factors); at the same time, the high concentrations present make possible large increases in active enzyme with a rapidity far in excess of that attainable by *de novo* protein synthesis.

The number of recognized enzymatically interconvertible enzyme systems is steadily increasing. Established and somewhat more tentative examples are given in Table 1.3. These enzymes are likely to play important roles in the regulation of their respective pathways. As with zymogen systems, the process of enzymatic interconversion allows a rapid switch from very low to high activity; this is, however, physiologically reversible, and, being intracellular, thereby conserves enzyme protein. This reversibility permits, for example, the synthesis and breakdown of food reserves to be tightly controlled in a manner that could neither be achieved so rapidly by *de novo* synthesis nor so completely by binding of activator or inhibitor molecules.

A number of non-enzyme proteins are also known to be subject to reversible covalent modification. These include certain ribosomal proteins and troponin, a component of the contractile system in muscle. The relative activities and importance of the 'normal' and phosphorylated forms is not clear, although troponin phosphorylation parallels the force of contraction in the isolated rat heart; evidence is accumulating that phosphorylation increases the sensitivity of troponin to Ca^{2+}.

In a few instances, enzymes may have two forms of differing activities, whose interconversion is mediated by specific small molecular weight ligands rather than enzymes. This has been shown for certain pyruvate kinase activities, acetyl CoA carboxylase and for glutamine phosphoribosylpyrophosphate amidotransferase, the first enzyme of *de novo* purine synthesis. These may perhaps be regarded as special cases where the ligand-induced transition between two conformers (e.g. R and T forms) is unusually slow.

The number of enzymes regulated by the binding of other, 'specifier', proteins is still small (Table 1.4), but may confidently be expected to grow in the near future. We may consider lactose synthetase as the best-known example. The A protein of lactose synthetase occurs naturally in the liver and mammary gland (during pregnancy). On its own, A protein is involved in glycoprotein synthesis catalysing the reaction:

UDP galactose + N-acetylglucosamine → N-acetyl lactosamine + UDP.

After parturition, B protein (α-lactalbumin) is rapidly synthesized in the mammary gland. This binds to A protein, suppresses its previous activity, and 'specifies' the new function of lactose synthesis [17],

UDP galactose + glucose → lactose + UDP.

(c) *Binding of effectors.* $[E]_{active}$ is frequently less than $[E]_{total}$ by virtue of the binding of specific inhibitors. Whether the inhibition is non-competitive (a physiologically infrequent event) or competitive, the proportion of the total number of enzyme molecules (i.e. $[E]_{active}$)

Table 1.4 Specifier proteins

Enzyme	Specifier	Action of specifier
Lactose synthetase A protein	Lactose synthetase B protein (α-lactalbumin)	Directs activity from glycoprotein to lactose synthesis.
RNA polymerase	σ factor	Specifies for discrimination for initiator-codon on DNA template.
Protein kinase	Cyclic AMP-binding protein (R protein)	Inhibits activity; dissociates from enzyme when cyclic AMP binds.
Glutamine synthetase adenylyltransferase	Adenylyltransferase activator (P_{II} protein)	Unmodified activator specifies adenylylation. Uridylylated activator specifies deadenylylation.

able to react with a fixed concentration of substrate is reduced, the more so at higher inhibitor concentrations. Conversely, this process may be reversed by the simultaneous presence of activator ligands. The proportion of $[E]_{total}$ which is denoted by $[E]_{active}$ is thus a function of the relative concentrations of specific activators and inhibitors. Many regulatory enzymes exhibit sigmoid rate response curves with increasing substrate concentration; the binding of effector ligands frequently alters the degree of such sigmoidicity, such that the effect of the ligand is markedly greater than that expected from enzymes which obey simple Michaelis-Menten kinetics. For details of the molecular processes involved in these interactions, the reader is referred to specialist texts [18].

(d) *Induction and repression.* This is the most obvious way in which enzyme activity is controlled *in vivo*, i.e. through the amount of total enzyme protein present. In contrast to (c) above, which is often termed 'fine' or 'acute' control, induction and repression constitute 'coarse' or 'long-term' control.

Since there is, under normal growth conditions, little enzyme degradation and protein turnover in prokaryotes, regulation of enzyme content in these organisms is very largely effected through changes in synthesis rate, and specifically through changes in synthesis rate, and specifically at the level of DNA transcription into messenger RNA (as, for example, in the *lac, his* or *ara C* operons [19]).

In mammals, control of enzyme concentrations is more complex. There is indeed evidence for control at transcription, but also at post-transcriptional events which include messenger RNA processing and polysome aggregation and activity. There is furthermore a growing suspicion (see 2.5.3) that control of enzyme degradation, possibly through specific energy- requiring processes, may be particularly important for many regulatory systems. Certainly the rates at which cell proteins turn over are very variable; in general regulatory enzymes exhibit shorter half-lives than do structural proteins and enzymes catalysing equilibrium steps (Table 1.5).

Table 1.5 Half-lives of intracellular enzymes in rat liver

Enzyme	$t_{1/2}$
Ornithine decarboxylase	11 min
δ-Aminolevulinate synthetase	1 h
Tyrosine aminotransferase	1.9 h
Tryptophan dioxygenase	2 h
Phosphoenolpyruvate carboxykinase	13 h
Catalase	30 h
Aspartate aminotransferase	60 h
Arginase	4–5 days

19

References

[1] Krebs, H.A. and Veech, R.L. (1969), In *The Energy Level and Metabolic Control in Mitochondria*, ed. Papa, S., Tager, J.M., Quagliariello, E. and Slater, E.C. Adriatica Editrice, Vari. pp. 329-382; Williamson, J.R., *Ibid*, pp. 385-400.

[2] Chappell, J.B. and McGivan, J.D. (1975), *FEBS Letters*, **52**, 1-7.

[3] Exton, J.H. and Park, C.R. (1969), *J. Biol. Chem.*, **244**, 1424-1433.

[4] Clifford, A.J., Rumallo, J.A., Baliga, B.S., Munro, H.N. and Brown, P.R. (1972), *Biochim. Biophys. Acta*, **277**, 443–458.

[5] Krebs, H.A. (1957), *Experientia* **16**, 125-132.

[6] Hales, C.N. (1966), *Essays in Biochemistry*, **3**, 73-104.

[7] Milstein, S. and Kaufman, S. (1975), *J. Biol. Chem.*, **250**, 4782-4785.

[8] Feliu, J.E., Aragon, J.J. and Sols, A. (1975), *10th Meeting of Fedn. of European Biochem. Socs., Paris, Abs.*, **846**.

[9] Chance, B. and Williams, G.R. (1956), *Adv. Enzymol.*, **17**, 65-134.

[10] Chance, B., Williams, G.R., Holmes, W.F. and Higgins, J. (1955), *J. Biol. Chem.*, **217**, 439-451.

[11] Williamson, J.R. (1966), *J. Biol. Chem.*, **241**, 5026-5036.

[12] Berneis, K.H., Pletscher, A. and Da Prada, M. (1970), *Brit. J. Pharmacol.*, **39**, 382-389.

[13] Warner, A.H. and McClean, D.K. (1968), *Develop. Biol.*, **18**, 278-293.

[14] Srere, P. and Mosbach, K. (1975), *Ann. Rev. Microbiol.*, **28**, 61-83.

[15] England, P.J., Denton, R.M. and Randle, P.J. (1967), *Biochem. J.* **105**, 32C-33C.

[16] Hess, B. (1973), *Symp. Soc. Exptl. Biol.*, **27**, 105-131.

[17] Brew, K. (1970), *Essays in Biochemistry*, **6**, 93-118.

[18] Gutfreund, H. (1972), *Enzymes: Physical Principles*, John Wiley, London.

[19] Lewin, B. (1974), *Gene Expression*, Vol. I, John Wiley, London.

Suggestions for further reading

Rolleston, F.S. (1972), *Current Topics in Cellular Regulation*, **5**, 47-75.

Sols, A. and Marco, R. (1970), *Current Topics in Cellular Regulation*, **2**, 227-273.

2 Practical aspects of metabolic regulation

2.1 General considerations

Chapter 1 has provided some brief indications of situations where practical problems can arise in the study of control mechanisms. This chapter deals with (i) the techniques which have been developed to overcome or circumvent such problems, (ii) the interpretation of experimental data, and (iii) areas where technical limitations impede further advance.

Ideally, the worker in this field would prefer to study a system which is, at the same time, both simple and chemically defined, and retains full physiological competence. Unfortunately, examples of this type are rare, and one is frequently faced with the alternatives of working with, for example, tissue extracts which provide clear, comprehensible data (sometimes!) but which are manifestly some distance from the natural state, and whole organisms with inter- and intracellular interactions, which at the very least, complicate quantitative interpretation. Some compromise is thus inevitable.

The choice of experimental system ultimately depends upon the type of information required. Whole tissue experiments will be necessary to reveal the extent of changes in flux rates through a pathway, to pinpoint rate limiting steps and to study changes in substrate and effector concentrations; use of crude homogenates might then permit kinetic evaluation of the individual enzymes under conditions where the possibility of artefactual modification is minimized; finally, purified enzyme studies can provide details of the molecular mechanisms of control. One cannot overemphasize that all of these approaches are necessary for a complete picture to be drawn, and that molecular details and interactions may themselves mean little unless it can also be shown that they occur in the physiological context.

The techniques for dealing with micro-organisms differ markedly from those used in mammalian studies. These differences arise largely from considerations of size and growth rate. Bacterial cultures rarely exceed 10^9 organisms per ml; protozoal cultures may be considerably less dense than this, even under optimal conditions. The intracellular water space in the densest cultures is thus less than 0.1% of the total culture volume. This means that total concentrations of metabolites in cells plus medium may be so low as to defy assay by conventional methods. The small size of most 'cells' again militates against the very rapid separation of 'cells' from medium for measurement of metabolite distribution under steady-state conditions. Nevertheless, prokaryotes especially may have several advantages. They may, for example, be grown in continuous culture under various environmental conditions or in large batches to yield appreciable weights of homogeneous 'cell' populations. Their rapid rates of division and mutation again make them ideal material for genetic experiments, which are very rarely possible in larger eukaryotes.

2.2 Animal preparations

2.2.1 Whole animals

The predominant characteristic of the whole

animal is that it is unarguably physiological. This advantage is offset by a number of other factors: (a) the system is very complex, and gives the experimenter little control over variations in hormone concentrations and other tissue interactions, (b) even when animals are from a single, inbred, strain there is great individual variability, so that the statistical validation of results may require the use of large numbers, (c) measurement of flux rates through metabolic pathways is usually very difficult, and (d) whole animals tend to be expensive. Nevertheless, the whole animal, and, particularly, the laboratory rat, is widely used in experiments designed to investigate the influence of various diets (or starvation) on gross metabolic parameters or enzyme concentrations. Such experiments may require up to several days for completion, and the whole animal remains the only 'preparation' which is 'viable' over such extended periods.

The effects of hormones may also be studied (or, indeed, minimized) in animals in which endocrine functions have been removed either surgically (e.g. hypophysectomy, adrenalectomy, pancreatectomy) or chemically (e.g. the induction of diabetes with alloxan or streptozotocin).

2.2.2 Isolated tissues
The isolated tissue again retains full morphological integrity, but is free from interaction with other organs. A few tissues, such as the rat epididymal fat pad, are small and thin enough for them to be incubated directly in medium since oxygenation is adequate. In many cases, however, the isolated organ is effectively oxygenated only by perfusion through the associated blood vessels.

For successful perfusion it is important that the time interval between removal from the animal and oxygenation with medium should be as short as possible to minimize damage caused by anoxia.

Problems can also arise where the effects of anaesthetics and/or the killing procedure persist in the tissue after removal from the carcass. These can frequently be overcome by including periods of pre-incubation or pre-perfusion (to establish steady-state conditions) in the experimental design.

A point often overlooked is that organs so isolated are necessarily denervated. This may have immediate consequences in that intracellular metabolism may be modified by sudden release (or inhibition of release) of transmitter substances. Another result has been that, until relatively recently, the coordination of metabolism by the nervous system has been a neglected research area.

2.2.3 Tissue slices
Tissue slices are now used less than formerly, having been replaced by the more physiological perfused tissue. In many cases it has been demonstrated that slices are irreparably damaged and exhibit metabolic rates much lower than expected. This is not a universal finding, however, and the slice remains a useful preparation for studying the metabolism of kidney cortex.

An apparent advantage of the slice technique is that it permits investigations to be performed on tissues which are too large or too difficult for successful perfusion, such as those from larger animals. Whether slices are truly valid preparations in these contexts remains to be demonstrated.

2.2.4 Isolated cells
The utilization of isolated cells is a relatively new technique which offers many advantages over others available. The most reliable methods of preparation involve incubation or perfusion of isolated tissues with collagenase. This breaks down the matrix so that individual cells may be released by subsequent gentle dispersal of the whole organ in buffer; cells are further freed from debris, etc., by decantation or sieving through nylon and gentle centrifugation.

Cell suspensions are homogeneous and permit multiple and reproducible sampling, an obvious advantage. They should, if correctly prepared, maintain rates of intermediary metabolism similar to those in the whole animal.

There is one serious problem which is often encountered; the effectiveness of collagenase treatment depends on the presence of a low level of proteolytic activity. This may degrade membrane-bound proteins including, especially, hormone receptors and transport systems.

2.2.5 Cell-free systems

This includes all systems where cellular integrity as evidenced by an intact plasma membrane has been destroyed. They may take the form of homogenates in buffer or may be 'reconstituted' by addition together of previously isolated components such as cytoplasm, mitochondria, nuclei or ribosomes. The major advantages of such systems are (1) the ease and reproducibility of preparations, (2) the relative simplicity, when compared to the whole cell, in respect of physical compartments, and (3) the absence of permeability barriers which might otherwise impede the effects of added compounds. Against these, one might argue forcibly that little remains of the nature of the original system, that organization is disrupted and diluted in media whose composition is often far from physiological, and that quantitative interactions between components *in vivo* are not necessarily easily reproduced by admixture *in vitro*. As elsewhere, the balance between these arguments depends primarily on the type of information sought. One can hardly deny the weight of data derived from the use of cell-free systems; nevertheless the literature contains a plethora of examples of unfounded extrapolations from homogenates and related preparations to the whole organism!

2.2.6 Isolated organelles

One approach to metabolic compartmentation is the study of the most obvious compartments in isolation. Developments in the field of density-gradient centrifugation in particular, now permit the separation, in good yield and purity, of most components previously identifiable only by microscopy. Most biochemical investigations have, however, been concerned with the mitochondrion and, to a lesser extent, the lysosome and nucleus. In particular, the sequence of electron-transport chain components, the transport of both anions and cations, and the integration of these processes, have become clearer from studies with isolated mitochondria. There are still, however, some problems in extrapolation. Ions which penetrate isolated mitochondria readily *in vitro* may not do so *in vivo*, owing perhaps to binding to other components or to competition for transport processes. Furthermore, populations of organelles are not necessarily homogeneous. Thus 'kidney mitochondria' include mitochondria from all sections of the renal tubule and other cells of the cortex and medulla — all known to be distinct biochemically — hardly a physiological mixture.

2.3 Preparations of specific tissues

2.3.1 Heart

The perfused rat heart is one of the most satisfactory *in vitro* tissue preparations. Substrates, hormones and oxygen are delivered in the physiological direction through an intact capillary network to the myocardium which is so close to histological homogeneity that one is effectively studying a single cell population. The organ is, furthermore, readily manipulated for subsequent metabolic assays. The older and simpler Langendorff preparation (Fig. 2.1) involves the cannulation of the aorta so that medium is forced through the coronary circulation by a combination of the perfusion pressure and contraction of the left ventricle. More recent preparations require cannulation of other cardiac vessels, a procedure which allows the experimental imposition of various 'work loads' to the aortic outflow.

2.3.2 Skeletal muscle

Although skeletal muscle constitutes some

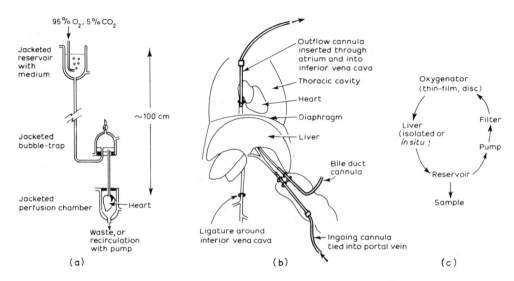

Fig. 2.1 (a) Simple flow-through Langendorff heart perfusion. Water at 37°C is circulated through the jacketed vessels. Medium may run to waste, be assayed directly for metabolites, or be recycled via a pump. (b) Positioning of cannulae for liver perfusion in the rat. The liver may then be removed from the rest of the animal or the whole animal may be used. The liver is then connected to the circuit shown in (c) in a thermostatted chamber.

70% of total body weight, technical difficulties in obtaining viable and useful preparations have prevented rapid advances in the understanding of muscle metabolism. The simplest source of striated muscle is the diaphragm which, in the rat, is of sufficient thinness for adequate oxygen diffusion through the surface; this allows incubation of whole diaphragms in medium in conical flasks.

Since contraction is the primary muscular activity, it is obviously not reasonable to attempt perfusion of entirely isolated muscle. Large amounts of muscle may be perfused, however, in the isolated hind-quarter preparation where medium is pumped into the abdominal aorta and returns through the ascending vena cava. Although the preparation is clearly by no means homogeneous, approximately 75% is muscle; the relative proportion of the total metabolic activity is probably higher still.

Lastly, much relevant information has been gathered from *in vivo* measurements of arterio-venous differences across muscular systems, particularly in man. Such experiments, for example, have clearly shown that a significant proportion of the carbon released during muscular activity is in the form of alanine and glutamine in addition to lactate.

2.3.3 Liver

The liver slice was for many years the standard preparation for investigations of liver function. The rates of urea formation are, for example, similar in the slice and *in vivo*. It is apparent, however, that the preparation is frequently far from physiological; slices leak enzymes and small molecular weight constituents so that adenine nucleotide levels may be very low indeed. Many of these problems arise from the larger than average size of the 'typical' liver cells (20–30 μm diameter); slicing thinly breaks many cells directly and 'shocks' others, whilst thicker slices may prevent adequate oxygenation.

The perfused liver is now perhaps the most widely used preparation. The organ is perfused, either *in situ* or in isolation, through cannulae in the hepatic portal vein (flow in) and in the inferior vena cava (flow out; Fig. 2.1). Many complex metabolic functions such as gluconeogenesis, albumin synthesis and lipoprotein and bile secretion are performed at physiological rates, testifying to the effectiveness of the preparation. Successful liver perfusion is, however, not easy and the number of livers that can be perfused in a short period is strictly limited. A second potential problem arises from the heterogeneity of the organ itself. Of the cellular material, some 90–95% is composed of parenchymal cells; these may be only 50–60% of the total number of cells since they are much larger than the phagocytic littoral (or Kupffer) cells. Whilst the parenchymal cells are generally gluconeogenic, even in the fed state, the littoral cells are normally glycolytic; this could provide a partial explanation of some claims of compartmentation of glycolytic intermediates in liver.

Yet more recently much attention has been given to isolated cells as tools for studying liver function. These are apparently homogeneous preparations of parenchymal cells, although there is some evidence to indicate that cells from different areas of the liver may differ quantitatively from one another. The possibility of large numbers of parallel incubations with these cells suggests that this preparation is a necessary complement to the perfused whole organ.

2.3.4 Kidney
The kidney is a visibly heterogeneous organ with clearly delineated outer cortex (approx. 80%) and inner medulla (approx. 20%). The metabolic activities of these regions are also different, e.g. the cortex is gluconeogenic whilst the medulla is actively glycolytic. Measurements of arterio-venous differences *in vivo* or of perfusate *in vitro* thus reflect the complex metabolic balance of the whole organ, and may be difficult to interpret.

Perfusion is nevertheless a useful technique for monitoring parameters of urine flow and composition.

Cortex slices exhibit metabolic fluxes close to physiological, and have proved overall to be the most useful preparation for biochemical investigations. Collagenase treatment of the cortex yields multicellular tubule fragments which are similar in activity to slices and which in many cases provide a more versatile system. It is apparent, however, that neither slices nor tubules represent homogeneous cell populations. Morphologically both contain proximal and distal tubule elements in addition to other cell types. Biochemical studies with 'purer' microdissected fractions reveal that there are major differences even between various portions of the kidney tubule. The preparation of pure cell types may depend on suitable disruptive procedures and the development of non-destructive gradient centrifugal techniques.

2.3.5 White adipose tissue
The most widely used adipose preparation is the epididymal fat pad. In a 150–200g fed rat the two pads weigh approx. 500 mg and are of sufficient thinness for adequate oxygenation in a simple flask incubation. The quantity of tissue, relatively high metabolic activity (in comparison with fat depots elsewhere), and *in vitro* 'durability' are undoubted advantages. The measurement of intermediary metabolites is, however, complicated by the small proportion of intracellular water (approx. 1.5% by weight), and frequently necessitates the use of fluorometric rather than simple spectrophotometric techniques. A further practical complication arises from the fact that the amount of stored triglyceride (by far the major constituent) varies widely between different physiological states. It can thus be to some extent misleading to express results in terms of the weight of tissue; since cellularity is more constant, DNA, tissue N or cell number may provide better indices.

Fat cells may be simply prepared by

collagenase digestion. Being less dense than aqueous buffers, they are easily freed from debris and other cell types by decantation. Once more, the homogeneity of such preparations facilitates the handling of large numbers of comparable samples.

2.3.6 Brain

Although brain is in many ways the most 'interesting' tissue, our understanding of its metabolism remains limited. The reasons for this are obvious enough. It is an organ of very complex function, which cannot always be clearly related to histological observation. This is discussed at length in a separate *Outline* [1]. Our present knowledge of brain metabolism is largely based on studies of arterio-venous differences across the organ and of slice incubations. A recent technique, 'freeze-blowing' (rapid pressurized removal and cooling of the organ, analogous to 'freeze clamping' of other tissues, see 2.4.2) now permits the measurement of in *vivo* whole-brain metabolites under controlled conditions. It should however, be emphasized that all measurements rely on a necessary, but almost certainly incorrect, assumption of the homogeneity of metabolite pools.

2.3.7 Islets of Langerhans

The Islets of Langerhans are small clumps of cells which constitute the endocrine pancreas, and whose major function is the synthesis and release of insulin and glucagon. Their very small total size in relation to the surrounding exocrine pancreas complicates investigation of their metabolism in the whole tissue. Islets may be isolated by collagenolytic digestion followed by microdissection or separation by density gradient centrifugation. Groups of islets may then be incubated as discussed for other isolated cell preparations. An alternative technique involves 'perifusion' whereby insulin release may be monitored continuously as the concentration of glucose (or other secretagogue) is varied.

2.4 Measurement of metabolites and their turnover

2.4.1 General problems

Although, by definition, the concentrations of metabolites within the cell do not change under steady-state conditions, individual compounds may be turning over very rapidly indeed. As examples, the phosphoenolpyruvate pool in aerobic heart muscle turns over completely in about 1 second, whilst the hepatic mitochondrial pool of oxaloacetate turns over some 500 times faster. The potential for rapid changes in total concentration when conditions are altered is therefore very great. Useful data will only be derived from accurate steady-state determinations so that it is very important that tissue or organism samples should be obtained and 'quenched' (i.e. all further metabolism blocked) as rapidly as possible to prevent any alterations being introduced by the experimental technique.

Accurate measurements can be further complicated by changes that occur even after 'quenching', e.g. (1) NAD^+ is destroyed in alkali, NADH in acid, whilst oxaloacetate and 1, 3-diphosphoglycerate are unstable at most pH values, and (2) residual activities of certain enzymes may remain; e.g. traces of adenylate kinase can result in a slow interconversion of ATP, ADP and AMP.

2.4.2 Quenching

The objective of quenching procedures is to secure the rapid cessation of metabolism, i.e. the inactivation or denaturation of enzymes. The most generally used method involves pH changes induced by addition of acid or, occasionally, alkali. Perchloric acid, $HClO_4$, is a suitable agent since it is a very strong acid, an effective protein precipitant, and can be simply removed after neutralization with KOH ($KClO_4$ is sparingly soluble). Trichloracetic acid, TCA, is also used but is less convenient because it can only be removed by repetitive extraction with organic solvent.

Organic solvents are effective denaturing agents at ambient temperature, but do not always act sufficiently rapidly for their use in metabolic experiments. They do, however, have one advantage in that the pH of the system remains at or near the original value; this can be important where the compounds under investigation are relatively unstable at extremes of pH. A good example is afforded in the early experiments on the carbon pathway of photosynthesis in *Chlorella* in which labelling patterns of intermediates were determined after short exposures to $^{14}CO_2$; algal suspensions were quenched in boiling methanol.

Where the experimental design involves incubation of thin tissues, isolated cells, cell-free systems or related preparations, almost instantaneous quenching may be achieved by simple addition of acid. In other situations where the preparation is larger, such as a whole perfused organ or tissue *in vivo*, metabolic activity must be first stopped by rapid freezing. The solid, powdered, tissue may then be subsequently extracted and denatured with acid.

Although liquid N_2 is sufficiently cold ($-196°C$), whole tissues freeze only slowly when immersed in it, because of the slow rate of thermal conduction through water (tissue 1 cm thick does not freeze entirely for approx. 20 seconds). The most satisfactory procedure is for the experimenter to clamp whole tissues (or appropriate portions) with 'Wollenberger tongs' whose jaws have been precooled in liquid N_2 (Fig. 2.2). The tissue is compressed into a flat 'pancake' and freezing is therefore facilitated (1 gm of tissue cools to $0°C$ in less than 100 ms, and to $-150°C$ in about 400 ms). These freezing times are remarkably short, but should nevertheless be compared with the rates at which metabolic profiles can change due to turnover (see 2.4.1), and with the rapidity of many physiological processes, such as the cardiac contractile cycle or general muscular activity (see 3.2.3).

When measurements of tissue concentrations *in vivo* are required, there is the further complication of the time taken to remove samples from the animal. The animal should optimally be killed instantaneously without prior stimulation which can affect the availability of adrenaline and other hormones in the blood. Anaesthesia avoids the latter, but frequently causes effects of its own. The time for killing to tissue freezing is usually 5–10 seconds. This necessarily includes a period of relative anoxia. Since some metabolites can change their concentrations dramatically in this time (5'-AMP may increase 5-fold in 10 seconds), conclusions drawn from such experiments should be tentative.

2.4.3 Assay of intermediary metabolites
The intracellular concentrations of glycolytic and citrate cycle intermediates, nucleotides, amino acids and their simple derivatives fall generally into the range 10^{-5} M to 10^{-3} M. If sufficient tissue is available, these compounds can mostly be assayed enzymically by standard spectrophotometric procedures, often involving the measurement of changes in pyridine nucleotide absorbance at 340 nm. Where concentrations lie below this range, or when tissue water samples can only be obtained at higher dilutions (e.g. adipose tissue extracts), a further 1–2 orders of magnitude of sensitivity can often be obtained with fluorimetry, again frequently with NADH or NADPH as fluor.

Certain metabolites cannot be assayed by conventional techniques or occur at such low concentrations as to be outside the normal sensitivity of optical techniques. The sensitivity may in many cases by increased by 'cycling' methods (Fig. 2.3). Possibly more generally, radioisotopic techniques may provide the necessary resolution. With microorganisms, or in isolated cell studies, it is often possible to label much of the intracellular metabolite pool by addition of labelled substrate; chromatographic separation, identification and radioactive counting can here provide simple, selective and sensitive assays for many constituents.

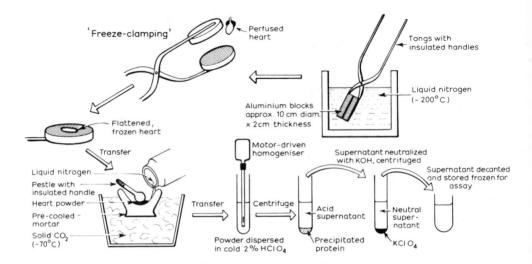

Fig. 2.2 Typical procedure for the preparation of extracts from perfused or isolated tissues. The tissue is rapidly frozen by pressure between two relatively massive aluminium blocks precooled to $-200°C$. The frozen 'pancake' is transferred either to a conventional mortar, as shown here, or to a stainless steel tubular mortar, for pulverizing. The temperature is maintained by direct addition of liquid nitrogen to the sample. The powder is dispersed rapidly in ice-cold $HClO_4$ by hand or mechanical homogenization, and the extract is finally neutralized as shown.

A second, somewhat more widely-applicable, technique is that of isotope dilution, frequently used for hormone determinations and increasingly for certain metabolites such as cyclic AMP (Fig. 2.4).

A number of yet more sensitive assay techniques are now beginning to be used more widely, and may permit a much greater understanding, particularly of minor, or 'specialist', pathways or metabolism. These include chemiluminescence (e.g. firefly and bacterial luciferases permit measurements of ATP and NADH respectively at the picomole and sub-picomole level) and mass spectrometric systems, which allow both separation and micro-quantitation of compounds in complex mixtures (e.g. gas and high pressure liquid chromatography coupled to high resolution mass spectrometers (GC-MS and HPLC-MS) and the use of integrated-ion current (IIC) techniques).

2.4.4 Compartmentation of metabolites

In mammalian systems, attention has been focussed almost exclusively upon two compartmentation problems, viz., the distribution of metabolites between the extra- and intra-cellular spaces, and between mitochondrial and extra-mitochondrial water. The possibility of uneven distributions between other organelles has as yet been little explored, but should not be discounted. Again, one should bear in mind the possibility of compartments other than those due to intracellular organelles (see 1.3.2). There are at present no generally applicable methods for resolving such compartmentation and this represents one of the major limitations to progress in many areas of metabolic regulation.

Total water in any one system may be simply measured using ^3H_2O; this is obviously freely in equilibrium with all 'pools'. The extracellular space can be estimated in a similar fashion but

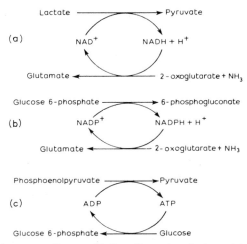

Fig. 2.3 Enzymatic cycling increases the sensitivity of spectrophotometric and fluorimetric assays by the inclusion of an amplification step. Thus in the presence of lactate, 2-oxoglutarate, NH_3, lactate and glutamate dehydrogenases and an appropriate buffer system, the rate of conversion of lactate and 2-oxoglutarate to pyruvate and glutamate is dependent on the concentration of added NAD^+ or NADH over a wide range (a). The amplification (i.e. pyruvate yield per NAD^+ or NADH added) may be up to $8000\ h^{-1}$ so that subsequent fluorimetric assay of pyruvate permits measurement of as little as 2×10^{-13} mol NAD^+ or NADH in the original sample. The technique may be extended in many ways, particularly by making use of the instability of NADH in acid and NAD^+ in alkali. Other cycling systems useful for the assay of $NADP^+$, NADPH and the adenine nucleotides are also shown above (b, c).

using a marker which is unable to penetrate cell membranes; [³H] inulin is a good example. In experiments with isolated mitochondria, 'contamination' of the pellet with medium components after high-speed centrifugation is often gauged with [¹⁴C] sucrose, which can penetrate the intermembrane space but not the matrix of the mitochondrion.

In many instances, however, it is not practicable to separate different cellular compartments. This is especially true in experiments designed to measure metabolites in whole tissues, either *in vivo* or *in vitro*, and where speed of quenching is of the essence. Since direct measurements of compounds in distinct compartments cannot be achieved, many attempts have been made to estimate concentrations indirectly. Thus, in rat liver, lactate dehydrogenase is exclusively cytoplasmic and probably catalyses an equilibrium

reaction. Since the K'_{eq} is known, the concentrations of lactate and pyruvate can be used to calculate the ratio of NAD^+ to NADH in the cytoplasm. Similarly, β-hydroxybutyrate dehydrogenase probably catalyses a reaction at equilibrium in the mitochondrion; measurement of acetoacetate and β-hydroxybutyrate permit calculation of the mitochondrial NADH/NAD^+ ratio (Fig. 2.5).

If the total malate and oxaloacetate concentrations are known, then it is possible to use the NADH/NAD^+ ratios in the two compartments to make some estimate of the distribution of these two metabolites across the mitochondrial membrane.

A further example is the calculation of the ratio of adenine nucleotides in the cytoplasm from metabolites confined to that compartment (Fig. 2.5). Such calculations are reliant, for their

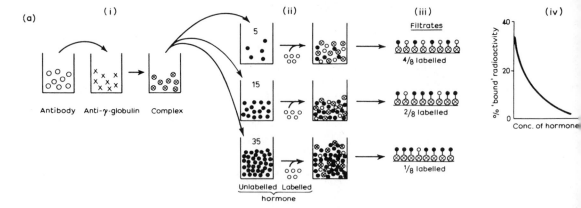

(a) 'Double antibody' radioimmunoassay, a method frequently used for peptide hormones.
(i) Hormone antibody mixed with anti γ-globulin fraction ('anti-antibody'). The complex formed is a microscopic precipitate. (ii) A known amount of the complex is mixed with standard known concentrations of unlabelled hormone (●), and a constant volume of labelled hormone (○) is added to all tubes (the label is often ^{125}I, a soft γ-emitter). (iii) After incubation, samples are filtered or centrifuged and the precipitate is counted. (iv) A standard curve is constructed from which the concentrations of hormone in test solutions may be calculated.

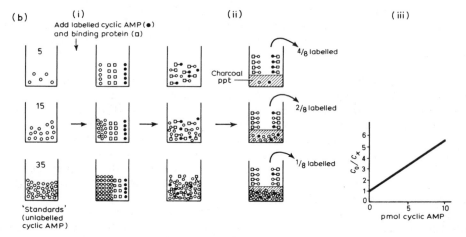

(b) Assay system for cyclic AMP. This method is also widely used for hormone assays where the hormone-antibody complex remains soluble and the hormone alone binds to the adsorbent.
(i) Unlabelled standard solutions are mixed with constant amounts of [^{3}H] cyclic AMP and limiting amounts of cyclic AMP binding protein (the R subunit of protein kinase). (ii) After incubation, charcoal is added, the tubes centrifuged and a fraction of the supernatant counted. (iii) A standard curve is constructed as before; C_0 — counts in sample with no added unlabelled cyclic AMP, C_x — counts in sample with specified amount of standard cyclic AMP.

Fig. 2.4 Isotope dilution assays.

accuracy, on a number of assumptions (e.g. free equilibration of metabolites within compartments, the maintenance of true equilibria, etc.) which are not necessarily always valid; indeed the arguments are often circular, assuming equilibration of certain intermediates between compartments to calculate distribution of others! Nevertheless, they are useful for example in indicating that the NADH/NAD$^+$ ratio in mitochondria is very considerably greater than that in the cytoplasm and that the ratios can probably be altered independently.

Attempts have recently been made to separate cytoplasm and mitochondria quickly enough for accurate direct measurement of the distribution of metabolites between these two compartments. One technique involves treatment of isolated liver cells with digitonin which causes rapid release of cytoplasmic, but not mitochondrial, constituents into the medium; the residual membrane plus mitochondria can then be spun down within 30 seconds [2]. This method is free from the assumptions of earlier, more indirect, procedures, but may still be rather too slow to give more than an indication of intracellular gradients.

2.4.5 Isotope experiments
Isotopic labelling is particularly useful in elucidating and evaluating the pathway by which a substrate is converted into its products. If to our suspected sequence A → B → C → D → E [^{14}C] A is added, then the specific activity of B will be equal to that of A, or lower if there is already some unlabelled B present; similarly, the specific activities of C, D and E will be the same or will fall at each successive step. If the specific activity of any intermediate (let us say C) is higher than that of its suspected immediate precursor (B), then one of two explanations may apply. In the first place, the sequence may not be A → B → C, but rather A → C → B. Alternatively, the specific activity of the pool of B converted to C may in reality be higher but appear lower due to dilution, during extraction, with a non-

exchangeable, and hence unlabelled, second pool of B.

The pattern of labelling in a product derived from labelled substrate may also indicate the pathway involved. Thus the labelling of glucose in the 1, 2, 5 and 6 carbons during synthesis from lactate-2-^{14}C indicates that equilibration of oxaloacetate with the symmetrical fumarate must have occurred at a rate rapid enough to permit randomization of the label.

Net flux through a pathway may also be deduced from labelling data, although great caution is needed in interpretation. [^{14}C] acetate is, for example, rapidly converted to [^{14}C] glucose in mammalian liver although no *net* flux is possible. The labelling pattern results from the fact that the two citrate carbon atoms lost as CO_2 in the tricarboxylic acid cycle are derived from oxaloacetate rather than acetyl CoA, and are thus unlabelled. After one 'turn' of the cycle, oxaloacetate will thus be labelled by [^{14}C] acetyl CoA and may of course give rise to [^{14}C] glucose.

Misinterpretation may also occur because of 'micro-equilibrium' considerations. When a reaction is not rate-limiting, there may thus be an appreciable back reaction (dependent on the absolute magnitude of the relevant rate constants). In such cases, labelled products can equilibrate rapidly with their substrates, thus giving the superficial appearance of net reversal, although the true flux may be in the opposite direction.

2.5 Measurement of enzymes and their turnover

2.5.1 General problems
Enzymes *in vivo* are frequently at concentrations some $10^4 - 10^6$ times higher than those used under standard assay conditions, are in environments vastly more complex, and may be part of either closely- or loosely-associated multienzyme complexes. In this event, it is perhaps surprising that activity measurements *in vitro* have been found to be generally consistent with overall physiological patterns.

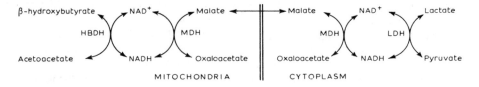

(i) *Cytosol NADH/NAD⁺ ratio*: assuming LDH to be in equilibrium, then

$$\frac{[\text{pyruvate}]\ [\text{NADH}]}{[\text{lactate}]\ [\text{NAD}^+]} = K_{\text{LDH}}, \text{ and thus } \frac{[\text{NADH}]}{[\text{NAD}^+]} = \frac{[\text{lactate}]}{[\text{pyruvate}]} \cdot K_{\text{LDH}}.$$

$K_{\text{LDH}} = 1.1 \times 10^{-4}$; both pyruvate and lactate may be readily measured, so that NADH/NAD ratios in the cytosol may be simply calculated.

(ii) *Mitochondrial NADH/NAD⁺ ratio*: as (i) but utilizing the HBDH equilibrium,

$$\frac{[\text{NADH}]}{[\text{NAD}^+]} = \frac{[\beta\text{-hydroxybutyrate}]}{[\text{acetoacetate}]} \cdot K_{\text{HBDH}}; K_{\text{HBDH}} = 4.9 \times 10^{-2}.$$

(iii) *Cytosol [ATP]/[ADP] [Pᵢ]*: if both of the following reactions are at equilibrium,

glyceraldehyde 3-phosphate + NAD⁺ + $P_i \rightleftharpoons$ 1,3-diphosphoglycerate + NADH (+ H⁺)

1,3-diphosphoglycerate + ADP $\rightleftharpoons$ 3-phosphoglycerate + ATP

then, defining K' as the overall equilibrium constant for the two reactions,

$$\frac{[\text{NADH}]}{[\text{NAD}^+]} = K' \cdot \frac{[\text{glyceraldehyde 3-phosphate}]}{[\text{3-phosphoglycerate}]} \cdot \frac{[\text{ADP}] [P_i]}{[\text{ATP}]}$$

Combining with (i), we obtain

$$\frac{[\text{lactate}]}{[\text{pyruvate}]} = \frac{K'}{K_{\text{LDH}}} \cdot \frac{[\text{glyceraldehyde 3-phosphate}]}{[\text{3-phosphoglycerate}]} \cdot \frac{[\text{ADP}] [P_i]}{[\text{ATP}]}$$

Since all these reactions are confined to the cytosol, indications of adenine nucleotide phosphorylation in that compartment may be obtained from measurements of the other metabolites in the overall equilibrium. $K' = 5.9 \times 10^{-6}$.

Fig. 2.5 Intracellular compartmentation. Calculation of cytoplasmic and mitochondrial redox states. HBDH — β-hydroxybutyrate dehydrogenase; LDH — lactate dehydrogenase; MDH — malate dehydrogenase.

Other factors may also be significant. Conventional Michaelis-Menten kinetic analyses do not, for example, apply where the concentration of enzyme is as great or greater than that of its substrate(s). Again, it is often difficult to assess the relevance of subunit association-dissociation phenomena in the whole tissue. Errors in interpretation may, however, arise from simpler factors. The process of extraction necessarily removes weakly-bound cofactors which must be replaced for maximal activity. For example, this seems a particularly awkward problem with pteridine-linked enzymes where enzyme activity may be fully expressed only with the natural cofactor, which is often not easily identifiable; the substitution of even closely-related compounds *in vitro* frequently results in sub-optimal activities. In the case of

Table 2.1 'Marker' enzymes for various organelles. Note that not all tissues will exhibit all enzyme activities, e.g. glucose 6-phosphatase is not found in non-gluconeogenic tissues. These distributions are derived from work with rats and related species; they do not necessarily hold for all species.

Plasma membrane:	$5'$-nucleotidase
Nucleus:	NAD pyrophosphorylase
Lysosomes:	Acid phosphatase, β-glucuronidase
Peroxisomes:	Catalase
Microsomes:	Glucose 6-phosphatase, Cytochrome P_{450}
Mitochondria	
outer membrane:	Monoamine oxidase, Kynurenine hydroxylase
between membranes:	Adenylate kinase
inner compartment:	Citrate cycle enzymes
	Glutamate dehydrogenase
	β-hydroxybutyrate dehydrogenase
	Ornithine transcarbamylase
	Pyruvate carboxylase
Cytosol:	Glycolytic enzymes
	Pentose phosphate pathway
	Arginase and others

interconvertible enzymes, it is important to emphasize again that substantial inaccuracy can arise because of changes in expressed activity during extraction in conventional buffers. As with metabolites, quenching must be rapid. Since acid is clearly inappropriate, the activities of the interconverting enzymes must be blocked with suitable inhibitors. For example, the relative proportions of phosphorylases a and b in muscle may be measured in extracts in buffers containing both fluoride and EDTA; the former inhibits phosphorylase a phosphatase and the latter, by chelating Mg^{2+}, phosphorylase b kinase. The two forms of the enzyme are thus 'frozen' in the ratio present *in vivo*. Experimental V_{max} determinations enable easy monitoring of changes in catalytic efficiency occasioned by hormonal or other effectors, but can obscure changes in K_m for specific substrates. Thus, the K_m of cyclic AMP phosphodiesterase for the nucleotide is lowered in liver following exposure to insulin, although the V_{max} remains unchanged.

2.5.2 Compartmentation of enzymes
Measurement of the distribution of enzymes between the various cell compartments is very much easier than that of intermediates, since enzyme concentrations are stable over longer time periods. There are, however, some practical problems. Fractionation of cells into their component organelles is rarely a 'clean' process; most fractions are contaminated with each other to some degree. This contamination can be allowed for, if the activities of enzymes of known cellular localization are measured at the same time as those of the enzymes under study. Some known examples of enzyme distribution are given in Table 2.1. The possibility that some enzymes are loosely associated with membrane structures and are released during homogenisation, thereby appearing in the soluble fractions – or that soluble proteins become abnormally associated with particles – should not be disregarded; practical proof of either is difficult without specialized histochemical techniques.

2.5.3 Measurement of enzyme turnover

In higher organisms, protein is constantly synthesized and degraded, the steady-state concentration being controlled by the relative rates of these two processes. Many experiments have been performed to show that individual enzyme activities are altered, sometimes very drastically, by changes in conditions (e.g. starvation, diabetes, steroid treatment, etc.). Measurements of activity alone, however, provide poor indices of the relative rates of synthesis and breakdown; in some cases, it is clear that activity changes *in vitro* are not parallelled by alterations in protein concentration, i.e. specific activity is not always a constant property.

A better method is that of immunoprecipitation. The enzyme is labelled with a 'pulse' of radioactive precursor, often an amino acid, and is then isolated by precipitation from crude tissue extracts with specific antibody (Fig. 2.6). Such techniques depend upon the ease of prior purification of the enzyme to homogeneity in sufficient quantity (to be used for raising antibodies), the antigenicity of the enzyme and the specificity of the antibody; these considerations remain important limitations in this field.

The form of labelled precursor is of importance. The higher potential specific activity of ^{3}H as compared to ^{14}C has led to the general use of [^{3}H]leucine in these studies. Nevertheless, in liver, at least, leucine is little degraded, and there is a strong probability that [^{3}H]leucine released during turnover may be reincorporated into protein rather than lost; this effect would tend to make protein half-lives appear longer than they actually are. This problem can be surmounted in liver with [^{14}C-guanidino]arginine (or $H^{14}CO_3^-$, which gives rise to this) instead; ^{14}C is then released as urea during turnover and cannot be reincorporated. Experiments with this latter method have in many cases revealed shorter half-lives than hitherto suspected, and thus tend to confirm that substantial reincorporation of much amino acid occurs. A third method, which also takes the reutilization problem into account and is applicable to many tissues uses both [^{3}H] and [^{14}C]leucine injected at different times. The ratio of ^{14}C to ^{3}H in isolated enzyme can then be related to the half-life.

Attempts to analyse the relative roles of transcription, translation and other processes in enzyme synthesis have frequently depended on the use of specific blocking agents. Actinomycin has been a widely used transcriptional inhibitor, but may give misleading data because of its 'side effects' — appetite and digestion are impaired, and the blocking of ribosomal RNA synthesis leads to additional inhibition of translation. More selective as transcriptional blockers are α-amanitin, an inhibitor of nucleoplasmic RNA polymerase, and cordycepin (3'-deoxyadenosine) which interferes with the production and release of mRNA by the nucleus.

Puromycin was the first translation inhibitor used, but has fallen somewhat out of favour due to its relatively low potency and 'side effects', e.g. the structural similarity to cyclic AMP results in sustained hepatic glycogenolysis in rats treated with this compound. Cycloheximide, which inhibits the GTP-dependent translocation of ribosomal subunits, is both more potent and specific. Translation in both mitochondria and chloroplasts, which have many prokaryotic characteristics, is insensitive towards cycloheximide, but is inhibited by the antibiotic chloramphenicol.

More recently, the problems engendered by insufficiently specific blocking agents together with the discovery that most, if indeed not all, mRNA is characterized by terminal poly A chains have stimulated more direct measurements of specific mRNAs. Isolation of total mRNA is achieved through binding to cellulose or, better, to columns of poly dT. Specificity and quantitation are gauged by addition of such mRNA to reconstituted systems capable of active protein synthesis (e.g. reticulocyte lysate, wheat germ extracts). Incorporation of labelled amino acid into particular proteins

(a) *Necessary preconditions*
1. Purification of enzyme.
2. Check of enzyme homogeneity.
3. Preparation of antibody; check of specificity by double diffusion and sodium dodecyl sulphate gel electrophoresis.
4. Check of time-course of incorporation of injected label into protein for tissue under investigation; this identifies the time at which steady-state incorporation is reached.

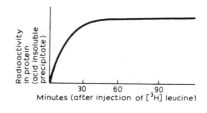

(b) *Routine procedures*
1. Group of animals injected with [^{3}H]leucine 60 min before killing and removal of tissue.
2. Tissue from each animal homogenised, centrifuged and the supernatants assayed for enzymic activity.
3. To an appropriate sample of each supernatant is added a slight excess of enzyme-specific antibody. After the necessary incubation period, the antigen-antibody complexes are precipitated by centrifugation, washed, reprecipitated and counted (A).
4. The supernatant from the first antibody precipitation is then treated with a second similar volume of antibody. Incubation and centrifugation are as before and the precipitate is again counted (B).
5. A sample of the original supernatant is treated with trichloracetic acid to precipitate total protein. This is washed, reprecipitated by centrifugation and counted (C).
6. 'A' includes the counts due to [^{3}H]leucine in the specific enzyme plus background due to adsorbed protein. This latter is assumed to be identical to the counts in 'B', so that 'A-B' represents counts in enzyme alone. 'C' gives the total counts in all soluble protein, so that $\frac{A-B}{C} \times 100\%$ indicates the relative synthesis rate of the specific enzyme as a function of total synthesis.

Fig. 2.6 Measurement of enzyme synthesis by immunoprecipitation. A typical protocol.

s again followed by immunoprecipitation (Fig. 2.6).

The rate of degradation of specific enzymes has as yet received less attention than that of synthesis. This is partly due to technical difficulties in following the disappearance of labelled proteins, but also to the lack of knowledge of the systems involved. Lysosomes certainly do degrade protein but it would be difficult to explain the great range of protein half-lives if this were the only mechanism (see Table 1.5). Certain enzyme groups such as the NAD$^+$-linked dehydrogenases and the pyridoxal phosphate-dependent transaminases may be degraded by specific proteases, but this again is probably a limited mechanism. There is, furthermore, some evidence that the break-down of regulatory enzymes (with short half-lives) is energy-linked and sensitive to agents such as cycloheximide. Clarification of these processes is needed before any quantitative appraisal can occur.

References
[1] Bachelard, H.S. (1974), Brain Biochemistry, Chapman and Hall, London.
[2] Zuurendonk, P.F. and Tager, J.M. (1974), *Biochim. Biophys. Acta*, **333**, 393-399.

Suggestions for further reading

General
Newsholme, E.A. and Gevers, W. (1967), *Vitam. Horm.*, **25**, 1-87.
Newsholme, E.A. and Start, C. (1973), *Regulation in Metabolism*, John Wiley, London.

Techniques
Bergmeyer, H.-U. (ed.) (1974), *Methods of Enzymatic Analysis*. 2nd English Edition, Academic Press, London.

Brolin, S.E., Borglund, E., Tegner, L. and Wettermark, G. (1971), *Analyt. Biochem.*, **42**, 124-135 (Chemiluminescent techniques).

Faupel, R.P., Seitz, H.J., Tarnowski, W., Thiemann, V. and Weiss, C. (1972), *Arch. Biochem. Biophys.*, **148**, 509-522 (Rapid quenching).

Lowry, O.H. (1973), An unlimited micro-analytical system. *Accounts of Chemical Research*, **6**, 289-293.

Lowry, O.H. and Passonneau, J.V. (1972), *A flexible system of enzymatic analysis*, Academic Press, London.

Mayer, J.R. and Boulton, A.A. (1973), Integrated Ion-Current Technique of Quantitative Mass Spectrometric Analysis. *Methods of Biochemical Analysis*, **21**, 467-514.

Mayer, S.E., Stull, J.T. and Wastila, W.B. (1974), Rapid tissue fixation and extraction techniques. *Methods in Enzymology*, **38**, 3-9.

Ross, B.D. (1972), *Perfusion Techniques in Biochemistry*, Oxford, University Press.

Scott, C.D. (1974), High pressure ion-exchange chromatography. *Science*, **186**, 226-233.

See also Methods in Enzymology, Vols. 32 and 39, (1975).

Compartmentation

Greenbaum, A.L., Gumaa, K.A. and McLean, P. (1971), *Arch. Biochem Biophys.*, **143**, 617-663.

Gumaa, K.A., McLean, P. and Greenbaum, A.L. (1971), *Essays in Biochemistry*, 7, 39-86.

Krebs, H.A. and Veech, R.L. (1969), In *The Energy Level and Metabolic Control in Mitochondria,* ed. Papa, S., Tager, J.M., Quagliariello, E. and Slater, E.C. Adriatica Editrice, Bari. pp. 329-38 (also Williamson, J.R., *ibid*, pp. 385-400).

Sols, A. and Marco, R. (1970), *Current Topics in Cellular Regulation,* 2, 227-273.

Srere, P. and Mosbach, K. (1975), *Ann. Rev. Microbiol.,* **28**, 61-83.

Enzyme Turnover

Goldberg, A.L. and Dice, J.F. (1974), *Ann. Rev. Biochem.,* **43**, 835-86

Katunuma, N. (1973), *Current Topics in Cellular Regulation,* 7, 175-203.

Schimke, R.T. (1969), *Current Topics in Cellular Regulation,* 1, 77-124

Schimke, R.T. (1973), *Adv. Enzymol.,* **37**, 135-187.

3 Examples of metabolic regulation in mammalian energy metabolism

3.1 Introduction

So far we have been concerned principally with outlining the various types of metabolic regulation and the means and approaches which are used in their investigation. Specific examples have been given but these have been restricted necessarily to isolated steps within metabolic pathways. This chapter attempts to discuss three complex areas in metabolic regulation at the level usually presented to the biochemist, namely the level of the intact tissue. All three areas are in the general field of energy metabolism and fuel interrelationships in animals. They are:—

1. fuel utilization in (heart) muscle;
2. conversion of carbohydrate into fat in adipose tissue;
3. carbohydrate synthesis in liver.

These processes play an important role in maintaining body homeostasis in the feeding-fasting and exercise-rest cycles which form the basic pattern of existence for most animals. Fig. 3.1 summarizes the major changes in metabolic flux occurring in animals during these cycles with emphasis on the areas to be discussed. On the whole, attention will be focussed very largely on the tissues of the long-suffering laboratory albino rat which is usually maintained on a stock high carbohydrate diet containing very little lipid. Probably conversion of carbohydrate into fat becomes less important as the proportion of fat in the diet is increased.

As will become evident, intensive research over the last 10–20 years has resulted in real progress in our understanding of the regulation of these three areas of metabolism. Further progress is limited in each case by the common problem of the compartmentation of metabolites either between mitochondrial and cytoplasmic compartments or between bound and free forms. Our knowledge of the regulation of glucose and glycogen metabolism in muscle is undoubtedly greater than that of other major metabolic pathways mainly because these processes occur predominantly in the cytoplasm and problems posed by compartmentation are fewer.

3.2 Fuel utilization in heart muscle

Metabolism of carbohydrate and lipid fuels by heart and other muscles is closely coupled to the energy needs of the organ. Changes in work load require changes in the rate of ATP supply and therefore changes in the rate of overall fuel utilization. Under anaerobic conditions, the only source of ATP is glycolysis and thus the only substrates that the heart can use are glucose and endogenous glycogen. However, the heart usually enjoys a plentiful supply of oxygen and can then oxidize a wide variety of fuels including glucose, lactate, fatty acids, ketone bodies, acetate and endogenous stores of glycogen and triglyceride. On the whole, the lipid fuels (fatty acids and ketone bodies) are oxidized in preference to the carbohydrate fuels (glucose, lactate) and this is important in conserving the latter in the fasting state. An outline of the pathways involved is given in Fig. 3.2.

When pyruvate derived from glycogen, glucose or lactate is being oxidized it is also necessary for reducing power generated as NADH by

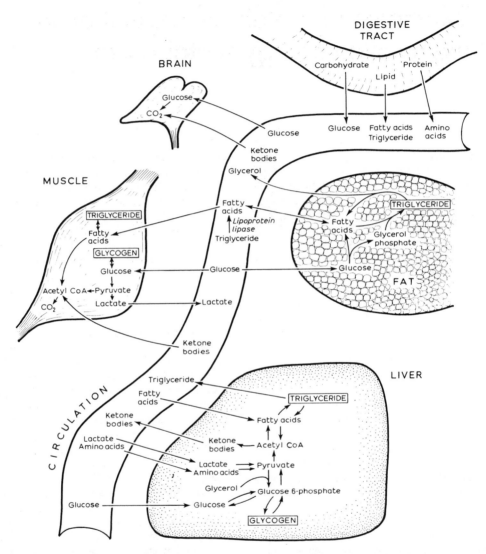

DIGESTIVE
TRACT

Carbohydrate   Protein
Lipid

Glucose   Fatty acids   Amino
Triglyceride   acids

BRAIN

Glucose
CO_2

Glucose

Ketone
bodies

Glycerol

MUSCLE

TRIGLYCERIDE

Fatty
acids

GLYCOGEN

Glucose

Acetyl CoA←Pyruvate
CO_2 Lactate

Fatty
acids
Lipoprotein
lipase
Triglyceride

Glucose

Lactate

Ketone
bodies

Fatty
acids   Glycerol
phosphate

TRIGLYCERIDE

Glucose

FAT

Lactate

CIRCULATION

Triglyceride
Fatty
acids

Ketone
bodies

Lactate
Amino acids

Glucose

LIVER

TRIGLYCERIDE

Fatty acids

Ketone
bodies   Acetyl CoA

Lactate → Pyruvate
Amino acids

Glycerol   Glucose 6-phosphate

Glucose   Glucose

GLYCOGEN

glycolysis to be transferred from the cytoplasm to mitochondria. Since the inner mitochondrial membrane is impermeable to pyridine nucleotides, this transfer must be accomplished by one of two indirect means. The so-called glycerol phosphate cycle is certainly important in insect flight muscle and perhaps some vertebrate skeletal muscle but the activity of the flavoprotein-linked mitochondrial glycerol phosphate dehydrogenase is rather low in heart muscle. Instead, the malate-aspartate cycle is probably the more important. (This cycle is the reverse of the one indicated in Fig. 1.4 for the transfer of reducing power out of mitochondria).

Fig. 3.1 Major interrelationships of energy metabolism in mammals.

Following a meal: carbohydrate, lipid and protein are broken down within the digestive tract, cross the intestinal mucosa and enter the circulation principally in the form of glucose, fatty acids, triglyceride (chylomicrons) and amino acids. These are stored in the peripheral tissues and liver very largely as glycogen and triglyceride. The major pathways operating under these conditions are probably:—

Muscle: glycogen synthesis from plasma glucose; triglyceride synthesis from plasma fatty acids partially derived by the action of lipoprotein lipase from plasma triglyceride (chylomicrons and very low density lipoproteins).

Fat: triglyceride synthesis from plasma fatty acids and triglyceride with glycerol phosphate derived from plasma glucose; on high carbohydrate diets fatty acids synthesized from glucose.

Liver: glycogen synthesis from plasma glucose and some amino acids; fatty acid synthesis from amino acids and glucose (dependent on diet); triglyceride synthesis from plasma and tissue-synthesized fatty acids (some triglyceride may be released as very low density lipoprotein).

During starvation: carbohydrate reserves (largely muscle and liver glycogen) are very much le.s than fat reserves (largely triglyceride in fat cells) and are conserved for essential uses. These include anaerobic glycolysis by red blood cells and (white) muscle and continuing oxidation by brain and central nervous system. Animals cannot convert fatty acids into carbohydrate. The major metabolic pathways operating under these conditions are probably:—

Muscle: lactate formation from glucose and glycogen; oxidation of fatty acids and ketone bodies.

Fat: triglyceride breakdown releasing fatty acids and glycerol.

Liver: triglyceride breakdown releasing fatty acids and glycerol; fatty acid oxidation to CO_2 and ketone bodies (released); gluconeogenesis and glycogen synthesis from amino acids, lactate, glycerol.

Brain: ketone bodies become progressively more important fuel than glucose.

During exercise:
Muscle: lactate formed from glycogen and plasma glucose (particularly in white muscle); glucose oxidation (but not in starved animals); fatty acid oxidation (and ketone body oxidation in starved animals).

Fat: triglyceride breakdown releasing fatty acids and glycerol.

Liver: triglyceride and glycogen breakdown releasing fatty acids and glucose.

During rest following exercise:
Liver: gluconeogenesis and glycogen synthesis from lactate and glycerol.

Muscle: glycogen replenished from plasma glucose.

Confirmatory evidence for a role for this cycle has come from the use of the transaminase inhibitor, amino-oxyacetate, which in heart muscle inhibits the oxidation of lactate and glucose. A major problem with the cycle is that all the reactions are apparently reversible yet it is believed that the cytoplasm is considerably more oxidized than the mitochondrial matrix on the basis of techniques such as those outlined in Fig. 2.5. It has recently been shown, however, that the efflux of aspartate from mitochondria is in exchange for glutamate plus a proton (Table 1.1) and is thus energy-linked.

3.2.1 Glucose and glycogen metabolism
Measurements of whole tissue concentrations of intermediates indicate that a number of steps in glucose metabolism are probably greatly

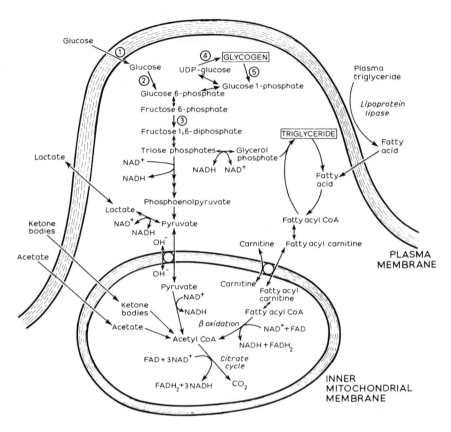

Fig. 3.2 Outline of heart muscle energy metabolism. The encircled numbers refer to enzymes and transport processes involved in the regulation of glucose and glycogen metabolism; the regulatory properties are summarized in Fig. 3.3 and Fig. 3.5.

displaced from equilibrium and are therefore potential sites for regulation. These include those catalysed by hexokinase and phospho-fructokinase and, under certain conditions, glucose transport, which are all thought to play important roles in the regulation of glucose uptake and phosphorylation. Properties of isolated preparations of heart hexokinase and phosphofructokinase and of glucose transport are summarized in Fig. 3.3.

Comparison of intracellular glucose concentrations with those in the perfusion medium indicate that glucose transport is stimulated by insulin and under anaerobic conditions. Accumulation of intracellular glucose under these conditions is indicative of the transfer of rate limitation of glucose metabolism from glucose transport to glucose phosphorylation by hexokinase. Hexokinase is inhibited by its product, glucose 6-phosphate, and this inhibition is non-competitive with respect to glucose. This means that changes in the activity of the next enzyme catalysing a non-equilibrium reaction, phospho-fructokinase, can regulate glucose phosphoryl-

Glucose transport and glycolysis
1. Glucose transport: activated by (i) insulin (mechanism unknown), (ii) anoxia, inhibitors of respiration, uncouplers (mechanism not established but probably related to changes in ATP: ADP: AMP).
2. Hexokinase: inhibited by glucose 6-phosphate (non-competitive with respect to glucose).
3. Phosphofructokinase: inhibited by ATP and citrate and activated by $5'$AMP, fructose 1, 6-diphosphate and phosphate and, to a lesser extent, ADP.

Glycogen metabolism

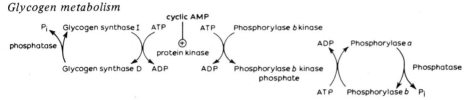

4. Glycogen synthase: I form is more active than D form in absence of glucose 6-phosphate. Glucose 6-phosphate activates both forms but its effect on the D form is inhibited (competitively) by phosphate and ATP.
5. Phosphorylase: activity of b form is increased by $5'$AMP but decreased by glucose 6-phosphate and ATP; except at high $5'$AMP concentrations b form always less active than a form. Phosphorylase b kinase; phosphorylation by cyclic AMP-dependent protein kinase lowers K_m for phosphorylase b; Ca^{2+} activates both phosphorylated and non-phosphorylated forms but the former is sensitive to lower Ca^{2+} concentrations.

Fig. 3.3 Summary of principal properties of enzymes and membrane carriers catalysing rate-controlling reactions in glucose and glycogen metabolism in the rat heart. Numbers refer to steps indicated in Fig. 3.2.

ation through changes in the glucose 6-phosphate concentration, and that this regulation will not be modified by the accumulation of intracellular glucose. This is important in a number of circumstances considered below, when changes in phosphofructokinase activity resulting from a change in the concentration of one or more of its many effectors are all important in initiating changes in glycolytic flux and glucose phosphorylation. Under these conditions inverse changes in glycolytic flux and the concentrations of glucose 6-phosphate and fructose 6-phosphate are observed. Most important in this context is the sensitivity of phosphofructokinase to changes in the adenine nucleotides, especially AMP, and in citrate. The step catalysed by pyruvate kinase is also displaced far from equilibrium but it seems rather unlikely, at least in muscle, that regulation of glycolysis is exerted

through changes in the activity of this enzyme. It would appear most likely that flux through this step is controlled very largely by substrate supply and thus by phosphofructokinase activity; studies on the isolated muscle enzyme have revealed little in the way of interesting properties except some inhibition by ATP.

Considerations of free energy changes, measurements of intermediate concentrations and properties of the enzymes concerned, all strongly point to regulation of glycogen breakdown and synthesis by changes in the activities of phosphorylase and glycogen synthase respectively. The regulation of these enzymes is complex and aspects are covered in detail in a companion volume [1]. Fig. 3.3 summarizes only aspects pertinent to the present discussion and is not complete. Both enzymes exist in two interconvertible forms, one phosphorylated and

41

the other non-phosphorylated, which have different maximal activities but, more importantly, have different sensitivities towards effectors. Removal of phosphate groups catalysed by a phosphatase leads to a form of phosphorylase (the b form) which is activated by AMP and inhibited by glucose 6-phosphate and ATP and which under most cell conditions is likely to be less active than the phosphorylated form (phosphorylase a). In contrast, removal of phosphate groups from glycogen synthase, catalysed probably by a different phosphatase, leads to a non-phosphorylated form of glycogen synthase (usually called the I form) which, under most cell conditions, will be more active. Glucose 6-phosphate can activate both forms but its effects on the D form are inhibited competitively by phosphate and ATP so that in the presence of one or both of these compounds higher concentrations of glucose 6-phosphate are required to stimulate the D form than the I form. Phosphorylation of phosphorylase b is catalysed by an ATP-linked specific kinase (phosphorylase b kinase) which is itself activated by Ca^{2+} in the range 10^{-8} to 10^{-6} M and by phosphorylation by the cyclic $3'5'$ AMP-sensitive protein kinase; phosphorylation of glycogen synthase is catalysed directly by the cyclic $3'5'$ AMP-sensitive protein kinase. On the whole, the complex regulatory properties of phosphorylase and glycogen synthase are such that conditions activating one will inhibit the other and vice versa, thus limiting the possibility of the futile cycle which would occur if both enzymes were active simultaneously. Recent studies by Cohen and his colleagues indicate that both phosphorylase b kinase and glycogen synthase may contain a second class of phosphorylation sites involving separate phosphatases and kinases. When these second sites are phosphorylated it appears that the enzyme activity may remain unaltered but that the susceptibility of the first class of sites to phosphorylation and dephosphorylation by the enzymes described alone may be altered. This form of regulation is considered in greater detail in the *Outline* written by Dr. Cohen [1].

The tissue concentrations of the three hexose monophosphates change in parallel, keeping the ratio of glucose 1-phosphate: glucose 6-phosphate: fructose 6-phosphate at about 0.5:10:2. This is consistent with the reactions catalysed by glucose 6-phosphate isomerase and phosphoglucomutase being very close to equilibrium. The size of the overall hexose monophosphate pool is presumably determined by the relative activities of phosphofructokinase and glycogen synthase, which regulate outflow from the pool, on the one hand, and hexokinase and phosphorylase, which regulate replenishment of the pool from glucose and glycogen, on the other. The activities of all four of these enzymes are affected by changes in the concentration of a constituent of the hexosemonophosphate pool (Fig. 3.4). Increases in the pool size may increase phosphofructokinase activity (activity increases sigmoidally with increasing fructose 6-phosphate concentration) and glycogen synthase (which is activated by glucose 6-phosphate) while inhibiting hexokinase and phosphorylase. There thus seems to be a basic system of regulatory mechanisms by 'feed forward activation' and 'end-product inhibition' which may act to keep the size of the hexose monophosphate pool within certain bounds and serve to integrate glycolysis and glycogen metabolism. Superimposed on this basic system appear to be specific mechanisms of regulation which are important in ensuring that appropriate responses are made in glucose and glycogen metabolism towards anoxia, insulin, adrenaline, fat fuels and changes in work load.

(i) *Anoxia.* If the supply to heart and other muscle is restricted, the rates of glucose uptake and glycogen breakdown are very markedly increased. Glycolysis is the only pathway able to form ATP from ADP and P_i in the absence of oxygen; under these conditions the end product of glycolysis is lactate so that NADH formed at glyceraldehyde 3-phosphate

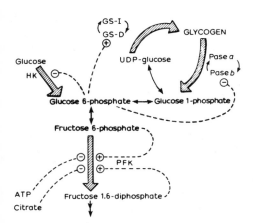

Fig. 3.4 The hexosemonophosphate pool and its interactions with hexokinase (HK), phosphofructokinase (PFK), phosphorylase (Pase), and glycogen synthase (GS).

dehydrogenase is utilised at lactate dehydrogenase, reforming NAD^+. The changes in glucose and glycogen metabolism probably involve parallel activations in glucose transport, hexokinase, phosphofructokinase and phosphorylase since the intracellular concentration of glucose is increased while that of the hexose monophosphate pool is decreased. The changes in activity of phosphofructokinase, hexokinase and phosphorylase can be explained rather satisfactorily in terms of the known properties of the enzymes and the observed changes in tissue metabolite levels. The mechanism whereby anoxia leads to increased glucose transport is not understood though it would seem rather likely that the increase is closely linked with changes in adenine nucleotides and especially AMP which occur under these conditions.

Activation of phosphofructokinase may be partially accounted for by the fall in ATP concentration observed in anoxia but probably more important is the associated rise in AMP. Heart and many other tissues contain high activities of the enzyme adenylate kinase (myokinase) which catalyses the reaction:—

$$2\ ADP \rightleftharpoons ATP + AMP\ (K'_{eq} \approx 0.5)$$

As this reaction is very likely to be close to equilibrium in cells and the ATP concentration is 30–100 times higher than that of AMP, a small decrease in ATP concentration will result in a much larger fractional increase in AMP. Typical values of ATP, ADP and AMP concentration in aerobic muscle are 10, 2 and 0.2 mM respectively which may change in anoxia to about 6, 2.2 and 0.4 mM respectively. Thus a 40% fall in ATP is associated with 200% rise in AMP. (Loss of total adenine nucleotide is because some IMP is formed under these conditions.) Regulation of phosphofructokinase through changes in the concentration of AMP can be considered to be an amplified variation of end product inhibition. If regulation were dependent directly on the concentration of the end product, ATP, a large drop in this metabolite would be necessary to initiate a large increase in glycolysis rate. This might result in the free energy available from the conversion of ATP to ADP and P_i being reduced below that sufficient to drive the essential energy-requiring processes in cells. Utilization of the adenylate kinase system to amplify changes in ATP concentration overcomes this problem; in particular it allows a large increase in flux through glycolysis to be achieved in anoxia with a relatively modest decline in ATP concentration. The concerted effect of the changes in adenine nucleotides and those of fructose diphosphate may ensure that there is a very rapid transition in phosphofructokinase activity from one steady state to another.

Acceleration of flux through hexokinase probably results from the reduction in glucose 6-phosphate concentration and is thus secondary to the increase in phosphofructokinase activity. Activation of glycogen breakdown may be due in part to some conversion of phosphorylase *b* to *a* but it seems largely to be the result of activation of phosphorylase *b* by the rise in AMP (an activator) and the decrease in ATP and glucose 6-phosphate (both inhibitors).

The key change then in anoxia is taken to be the fall in ATP which, because of adenylate kinase, is associated with a much larger percentage increase in AMP concentration. This increase then activates, in parallel, phosphofructokinase, phosphorylase b and maybe also membrane transport of glucose. The concentration of the hexose monophosphate pool falls, removing inhibition of hexokinase and phosphorylase b by glucose phosphate.

(ii) *Insulin and adrenaline.* Insulin increases glucose transport thereby causing accumulation of intracellular glucose and transfer of rate limitation of glucose uptake to glucose phosphorylation by hexokinase. Insulin also increases the synthesis of glycogen probably by causing a greater proportion of glycogen synthase to be in the more active, 'I', form. The mechanisms involved in both these effects of insulin are not understood and detailed discussion is beyond the scope of this book. Changes in muscle cyclic AMP do not appear to provide a satisfactory explanation of the hormone's effects on glycogen synthase (see also Section 3.3.5).

Adrenaline causes increased glycogen breakdown through conversion of phosphorylase b to a by the cascade of reactions initiated by the increase in cyclic AMP outlined in Fig. 3.3; increased glycolysis may be largely the result of the rise in the hexose monophosphate pool which follows.

(iii) *Fat fuels.* The rate of glucose uptake and glycolysis in the perfused rat heart is markedly decreased in the presence of fat fuels (fatty acids, acetate, ketone bodies). This is most clearly demonstrated in the presence of insulin when the rates of glucose uptake and glycolysis are reduced by 50–70%. Under these conditions intracellular glucose accumulates and the size of the hexose monophosphate pool is increased, indicating that the probable mechanism involves inhibition of phosphofructokinase leading to the rise in the hexose monophosphate pool and thus to inhibition of hexokinase. The factor responsible for the inhibition of phosphofructokinase was a mystery for some time since no changes in adenine nucleotides were evident. Then it was found that citrate was a potent inhibitor of phosphofructokinase and furthermore that the heart content of citrate ris when fatty acids or ketone bodies are being oxidized. Citrate thus appears to act as the signal which ensures that glucose metabolism is restricted when lipid fuels are available. In the heart, citrate can only be formed and metabolized in the mitochondrion and must be trans ported into the cytoplasm to inhibit phosphofructokinase; heart muscle mitochondria contai the necessary specific transporter for citrate (see Section 3.2.3).

(iv) *Work load.* When the work load of the perfused rat heart is increased, glucose and glycogen metabolism through glycolysis is increased almost certainly because glucose trans port, phosphorylase b and phosphofructokinase activity are all increased. However, the mechanisms involved have yet to be defined as no changes in adenine nucleotides are evident unless very high work loads are used. One possibility which will be raised again later is that changes in ATP and ADP concentrations and particularly AMP are occurring within each beat but that these changes are not picked up by current freeze-clamping techniques.

3.2.2 Pyruvate metabolism

Conversion of glucose and glycogen to lactate in muscle does not necessarily deplete body carbohydrate reserves because lactate may be used as a substrate for gluconeogenesis in liver and kidney (Cori cycle, see Fig. 3.11). However, conversion of pyruvate to acetyl CoA by the pyruvate dehydrogenase complex is a functionally irreversible process and represents real loss in body carbohydrate reserves in animals because they lack the capacity for synthesizing glucose from acetyl CoA. (This is

(a) Reaction sequence

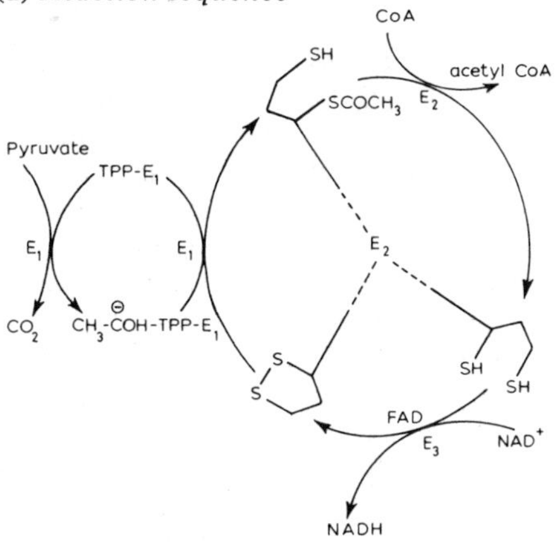

The complex (mol. wt. about 10^7) is composed of a core of 60 E_2 (dihydrolipoate transacetylase) to which is attached about 60 E_1 (pyruvate decarboxylase) and about 12 E_3 (dihydrolipoate dehydrogenase); E_1 is composed of 2 subunits, α and β. In the formation of acetyl CoA and NADH from pyruvate the lipoate group covalently bound to E_2 visits in turn active centres on E_1, E_2 and E_3, which transform the oxidized lipoate group first to acetyl hydrolipoate, then dihydrolipoate and thence back to the oxidized form. (TPP is thiamine pyrophosphate.)

(b) Regulation

(i) End product inhibition by increasing concentration ratios of acetyl CoA/CoA and NADH/NAD$^+$. Mechanism may be through a change in proportion of lipoate in the oxidized form.

(ii) Phosphorylation-dephosphorylation of the α-subunits of E_1. V_{max} of phosphorylated form is less than 1% non-phosphorylated form.

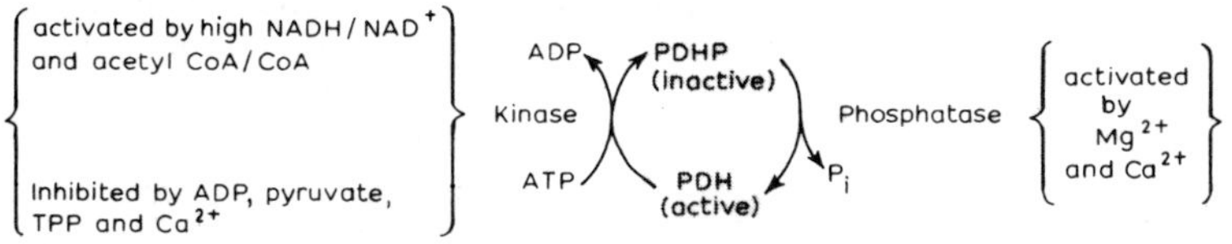

N.B. Cyclic AMP does not effect the activity of the kinase or any other component of the system.

Fig. 3.5 The mammalian pyruvate dehydrogenase complex.

accomplished in some plants and bacteria by the glyoxalate pathway.) Regulation of pyruvate metabolism by the pyruvate dehydrogenase complex is therefore of crucial importance in animals. In starvation in particular, it is essential that pyruvate oxidation in muscle is all but eliminated in favour of the oxidation of lipid fuels.

Individual steps catalysed by the components of the complex are summarized in Fig. 3.5a, which also outlines some of the basic architectural features of the heart complex. Two types of regulation of pyruvate oxidation by the complex have been described: end product inhibition

by acetyl CoA and NADH; and the interconversion of an inactive phosphorylated form and an active non-phosphorylated form (Fig. 3.5b). A likely mechanism of end product inhibition is that, in the presence of high ratios of acetyl CoA/CoA and/or NADH/NAD$^+$, the proportion of the lipoate groups bound to the transacetylase core which are in the oxidized form is greatly reduced, limiting the activity of E_1 (pyruvate decarboxylase). The complex in mammalian tissues contains an ATP-requiring kinase which is strongly bound to the transacetylase core and which phosphorylates a subunit (designated α) of the pyruvate decarboxylase components.

45

Removal of this phosphate and reactivation is catalysed by a phosphatase which is rather loosely bound to the complex. Studies of purified preparations and isolated mitochondria have shown that the phosphatase requires Mg^{2+} and is also activated by Ca^{2+} (10^{-8} to 10^{-5} M) and that the kinase is inhibited by ADP (competitive with ATP, pyruvate, TPP and Ca^{2+}). In addition, it has been found recently that the kinase is activated by high ratios of NADH/NAD^+ and this effect can be enhanced by high ratios of acetyl CoA/CoA [2,3]. Thus phosphorylation and inactivation of the complex may be promoted under conditions when end product inhibition occurs. A number of mechanisms could be suggested for the effects of acetyl CoA, CoA, NAD^+ and NADH on the kinase. One attractive possibility which is consistent with the likely mechanism of end product inhibition is that lipoate may act as the transmitter of these regulatory interactions. It is possible that, when the lipoate group is in the oxidised form, it is 'parked' close to the α-subunit of the decarboxylase (E_1) and inhibits phosphorylation by steric hindrance or similar mechanism (Fig. 3.5a). Then conversion of the lipoate group to its reduced or acetylated forms in the presence of NADH and acetyl CoA may result in the transfer of the group to sites on E_3 or E_2 and lead to the observed increase in kinase activity [2].

Studies with isolated mitochondria have shown that the entire pyruvate dehydrogenase complex including its kinase and phosphatase are located within the inner mitochondrial membrane. The location of pyruvate dehydrogenase presents real problems in the identification of mechanisms involved in alterations in its activity because direct measurements of the concentration of substrates and effectors in the mitochondrial matrix within a whole tissue preparation are not generally feasible with current techniques. Similar problems will recur throughout this chapter. Changes in tissue concentration of glycolytic intermediates are probably a reasonable reflection of changes in the cytoplasmic compartment because these intermediates are largely located in that compartment. It is clearly rather more hazardous to use whole tissue measurements as an indication of changes in the mitochondrial concentration of intermediates since the mitochondrial matrix is only 15–20% of the heart intracellular volume and the concentration of most intermediates is unlikely to be the same on both sides of the inner mitochondrial membrane.

The rate of pyruvate oxidation is near zero in hearts oxidizing fat fuels (fatty acids, ketone bodies, acetate). This inhibition can be partially accounted for by a decrease in the proportion of the complex in its active (non-phosphorylated) form from about 25 to 10%. The simplest hypothesis at present is that when fat fuels are being oxidized the mitochondrial concentration ratio of acetyl CoA/CoA and possibly also NADH/NAD^+ is increased and that this results in suppression of pyruvate oxidation by a linked combination of end-product inhibition and increased kinase activity. The whole tissue concentration ratio of acetyl CoA/CoA rises rapidly by some 50-fold after the onset of the oxidation of fat fuels.

Further consideration of the role of the other effectors of the phosphatase and kinase is given in the Section (3.3.2) concerned with the hormonal regulation of the complex in adipose tissue. However, the possible role of changes in the mitochondrial concentration ratio of ATP/ADP should be noted. A fall in this ratio will inhibit the kinase and cause activation of the complex. However, a fall in the ATP/ADP ratio may also be associated with a proportionally larger fall in the NADH/NAD^+ ratio because of the relationship of these ratios one to another through the respiratory chain. Rates of pyruvate oxidation may therefore be geared to the needs of respiration not so much by changes in the mitochondrial concentration ratio of ATP/ADP directly but through the larger changes in NADH/NAD^+ ratio which may result from changes in the ATP/ADP ratio. Similar amplification of changes in cytoplasmic ATP/ADP ratios appears to be brought about by adenylate kinase (see above, Section 3.2.1).

3.2.3 Regulation of citrate cycle and fatty acid oxidation

The identification of regulatory sites in the citrate cycle is difficult. Studies on the properties of isolated enzymes suggest three candidates:—

(i) Citrate synthase: first step in cycle but activity high and K_m for substrates, acetyl CoA and oxaloacetate, low; however, inhibited by ATP and to a lesser extent other adenine nucleotides (competitive with acetyl CoA) and by citrate (competitive with oxaloacetate) which may greatly increase apparent K_m in situ.

(ii) NAD$^+$-dependent isocitrate dehydrogenase: ADP activates (lowers K_m for isocitrate). NADH and ATP inhibit (largely competitive with NAD$^+$). (iii) Oxoglutarate dehydrogenase: like pyruvate dehydrogenase, very large —ve free energy change and inhibited by high ratios of NADH/NAD$^+$ and succinyl CoA/CoA.

Unfortunately it is not possible by measurement of whole tissue concentrations of intermediates to ascertain with certainty whether any of these wholly mitochondrial steps are close to equilibrium and therefore unlikely to be regulatory. The proportional distributions of citrate, isocitrate. oxoglutarate, oxaloacetate, the CoA derivatives and NAD$^+$ and NADH between mitochondria and cytoplasm are all unknown and mass-action ratios for the mitochondrial compartment cannot be calculated with any confidence. In addition, oxaloacetate presents further difficulties because of its instability and very low concentrations. An alternative approach for the identification of non-equilibrium reactions is the study of the time courses of specific activities of intermediates immediately following introduction of a [^{14}C] labelled substrate. In the perfused heart, following introduction of [^{14}C] acetate, the specific activities of acetyl CoA and acetylcarnitine rise quickly but that of citrate

rises much more slowly and at a rate consistent with there being no back rate in the citrate synthase reaction. Labelling of other intermediates in the cycle is consistent with a back reaction of about 50% of the forward rate for the isocitrate dehydrogenase step and probably no back reaction at oxoglutarate dehydrogenase. These findings suggest that regulation of the citrate cycle could be exerted at citrate synthase and oxoglutarate dehydrogenase but not at NAD$^+$-isocitrate dehydrogenase. These conclusions are based on calculations which assume single pools of intermediates, i.e. that cytoplasmic and mitochondrial pools are in isotopic equilibrium or that the cytoplasmic pool is negligible in size. They do, however, provide a possible explanation for the time course of changes in concentrations seen in citrate cycle intermediates following the onset of oxidation of acetate or other fat fuels. Thus, following addition of acetate to perfusion media, the heart concentration of acetyl CoA rises within a few seconds and then over a period of the next five minutes there is a slow rise in citrate which is accompanied by parallel rises in isocitrate, oxoglutarate and glutamate and falls in aspartate and to some extent malate. This pattern is consistent with regulation at citrate synthase and oxoglutarate dehydrogenase. The rise in acetyl CoA would appear to increase flux through citrate synthase so that in the transient period the rate through the segment oxaloacetate to oxoglutarate is faster than the rate through the segment oxoglutarate to oxaloacetate which is limited by the activity of oxoglutarate dehydrogenase. This temporary 'dislocation' or 'unspanning' of the cycle would then explain the observed transfer of carbon from one half of the cycle (malate, aspartate) to the other half (citrate, isocitrate, oxoglutarate).

A consistent and fairly satisfactory sequence of events can now be proposed following onset of the oxidation of fat fuels. The oxidation results in a sharp rise in acetyl CoA which is important in causing the near immediate inhibition of pyruvate oxidation. The rise in acetyl

CoA also initiates changes in the citrate cycle which lead to an increase in the citrate concentration over the next five minutes causing parallel and progressive inhibition of phosphofructokinase and therefore glycolysis during the first few minutes of fat fuel oxidation. This must involve transfer of citrate from mitochondria to the cytoplasm most probably via the transporter which exchanges citrate for malate and which is present in heart mitochondria. A number of problems remain. For example, the transfer of reducing power from the cytoplasm to mitochondria is greatly diminished but it is not at all clear how this is achieved; it may be because the transfer of aspartate and/or malate across the mitochondrial membrane is inhibited. Such inhibition may also provide some explanation for the lag in the rise in citrate since most of the carbon may be derived from extramitochondrial aspartate. It is also not easy to fit in all the changes observed with dichloracetate (see next section).

The most fundamental problem, though, is the lack of any concrete understanding of the mechanisms which ensure that the production of mitochondrial reducing power by the citrate cycle, β-oxidation and pyruvate dehydrogenase is at a rate appropriate for the ATP needs of the heart. When the work load of the perfused heart is increased, the rate of oxygen consumption and therefore ATP turnover may be increased 2—3 fold. There are matching increases in flux through β-oxidation and citrate cycle and pyruvate dehydrogenase — but what causes these increases? Measurements of whole tissue concentrations yield no clues as few, if any, changes are found even in the adenine nucleotides. It is likely that important changes are occurring in the mitochondrial concentration ratios of ATP/ADP and NADH/NAD$^+$ but that these are not evident using freeze clamping techniques. One reason may be that the ATP utilization by muscle contraction is occurring only during contraction (systole) which represents about 40% of the cardiac cycle of 250 milliseconds. Thus concentration changes may be occurring

within each beat and are not observed because freeze clamping is at random times during the cardiac cycle and in any case freezing probably takes 100 milliseconds or more. On present evidence, the most likely hypothesis is that changes in the mitochondrial concentration ratio of NADH/NAD$^+$ are the all-important link between the oxidative pathways and respiration. As mentioned before, an increase in the NADH/NAD$^+$ ratio will result in inhibition of pyruvate dehydrogenase. It may also lead to inhibition of flux through the citrate cycle by causing reductions in the concentration of oxaloacetate and oxoglutarate (assuming malate dehydrogenase and isocitrate dehydrogenase catalyse equilibrium reactions in mitochondria) thus possibly limiting flux through citrate synthase and oxoglutarate dehydrogenase; this latter enzyme is also inhibited directly by a rise in NADH/NAD$^+$ ratio. Studies on changes in isolated rat heart mitochondria on addition of ADP support this view [3] but unfortunately it will remain a speculative hypothesis until methods are devised for the continuous monitoring of mitochondrial changes in NADH and adenine nucleotides within the intact heart during the cardiac cycle. Techniques involving firing 'silver bullets' filled with liquid N_2 at beating hearts to coincide with predetermined stages in the cardiac cycle have been devised recently and used to demonstrate that there are inverse changes in the concentrations of cyclic AMP and GMP within cardiac cycles [4,5], but this technique can only yield information about changes in whole tissue contents.

Very little is known about the regulation of fatty acid oxidation. The rate of supply of fatty acids from exogenous sources and endogenous triglyceride is an important factor but mechanisms must also be present to ensure integration of the rate of β-oxidation to the respiratory chain and to other oxidative metabolism. Obvious possibilities include regulation by CoA availability since much of the mitochondrial CoA pool is probably present as acetyl CoA when fat fuels are oxidized and regulation by the NADH/NAD$^+$ ratio exerted at the hydroxyacyl CoA dehydrogenase step.

3.2.4 Use of specific inhibitors to explore interactions of metabolism in the heart

Important confirmatory evidence for proposed regulatory mechanisms can sometimes be obtained from the use of specific inhibitors which perturb metabolism in a hopefully defined manner.

(i) *Fluoroacetate* [6]. This is converted in heart and other tissues to fluorocitrate, a very potent inhibitor of aconitate hydratase. In the heart, fluorocitrate leads to an increase in the concentration of citrate which is accompanied by a marked diminution in the rate of glycolysis and a concomitant increase in the hexosemonophosphate pool. This supports the suggested role of citrate in the regulation of glycolysis through its inhibitory effects on phosphofructokinase.

(ii) *Bromofatty acids* [7]. These fatty acids are thought to act by being first converted to their acyl CoA derivatives which are very potent inhibitors of the extramitochondrial carnitine fatty acyltransferase involved in the transfer of fatty acyl groups into mitochondria. Hearts from alloxan-diabetic rats have greatly reduced rates of glycolysis and pyruvate oxidation associated with high rates of oxidation of fatty acids derived from endogenous triglyceride; these correlate with increases in tissue citrate and acetyl CoA and changes in glycolytic intermediates consistent with inhibition of phosphofructokinase. However, in the presence of bromostearate, glucose utilization is increased while that of fatty acids is diminished to rates found in hearts of normal animals. Moreover the tissue contents of citrate, acetyl CoA and glycolytic intermediates also revert to normal which is strong evidence for the suggested roles of acetyl CoA and citrate in the regulation of

glucose and pyruvate metabolism.

(iii) *Dichloracetate* [8]. This is an inhibitor of pyruvate dehydrogenase kinase (perhaps because it is an analogue of pyruvate) and it causes the pyruvate dehydrogenase complex in heart muscle and other tissues to be converted largely to the active non-phosphorylated form. Addition of the inhibitor to hearts from alloxan-diabetic rats or hearts from normal rats perfused with fat fuels leads to greatly increased rates of glycolysis and pyruvate oxidation and inhibition of the oxidation of fat fuels. These changes are associated with a marked reduction in citrate concentration, again supporting the role of citrate in the regulation of glycolysis. However, the tissue content of acetyl CoA is not markedly decreased and thus the mechanisms which lead to this decrease in citrate concentration remain to be defined as do also the means whereby the oxidation of fat fuels is reduced under these circumstances.

3.3 Conversion of carbohydrate into fat in adipose tissue

3.3.1 General aspects of adipose tissue metabolism

Most triglyceride in animals is stored in fat cells of white adipose tissue. The metabolism of this tissue (Fig. 3.6) is almost entirely concerned with the synthesis of fatty acids and their storage as triglyceride following feeding and with the release of fatty acids from triglyceride during fasting or exercise. (Animals also contain brown adipose tissue which is capable of oxidizing fatty acids at high rates and generating heat. This tissue is important in thermogenesis in hibernating animals and the neonates of many species including humans.) Regulation of the major pathways in adipose tissue involves long term as well as acute types of control and is probably initiated primarily by changes in the plasma concentration of hormones. Adipose tissue is sensitive to a remarkably wide spectrum of hormones

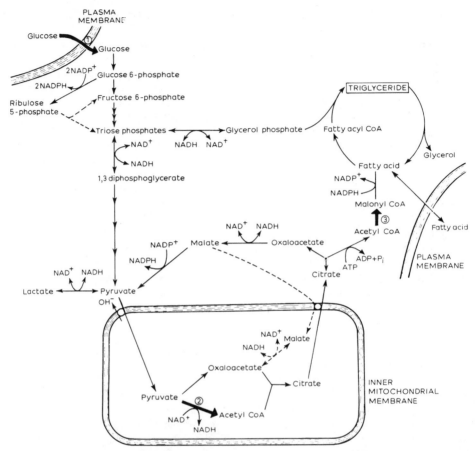

Fig. 3.6 Outline of the major pathways in rat epididymal adipose tissue. Steps which appear to be principally involved in the acute regulation of the conversion of glucose to fatty acids by hormones are (1) glucose transport across plasma membrane, (2) pyruvate dehydrogenase (intramitochondrial) (3) acetyl CoA carboxylase (cytoplasmic).

and studies on this tissue have been generally directed at understanding the mechanisms whereby hormones regulate its metabolism. Most studies have been carried out with the rat epididymal fat pad or fat cells isolated from pads by collagenase digestion.

The following sections will be concerned with the long term and acute regulation of the conversion of carbohydrate into triglyceride. But first a few words about the hormonal regulation

of the breakdown of triglyceride to release fatty acids and glycerol. Regulation appears to be exerted through changes in the activity of triglyceride lipase. This enzyme is activated by phosphorylation by protein kinase. Acceleration of lipolysis (triglyceride breakdown) by a number of hormones including adrenaline, glucagon and ACTH appears to be brought about by the interaction of these hormones with specific receptors on the outside of the fat cells leading to activation of adenyl cyclase in the plasma membrane and thus to increased cell cyclic $3'5'$ AMP and activation of protein kinase. Insulin inhibits lipolysis but the precise mechanism is not established. There is much controversy over the consequences of insulin binding to specific membrane receptors; in particular whether or not this event directly inhibits adenyl cyclase. Lipolysis is also subject to long-term regulation, for example in starvation. This may involve the combined actions of growth hormone and glucocorticoids since prolonged incubation of adipose tissue with both hormones increases lipolysis. This increase may be blocked if protein synthesis inhibitors are added throughout, thereby suggesting that induction of one or more enzymes is involved.

3.3.2 Pathways involved in fatty acid synthesis from glucose

The conversion of glucose into fatty acids in adipose tissue is easily demonstrated, and indeed measured, using [U-^{14}C] glucose; some of the important details of the pathways involved have, however, been difficult to define with certainty.

The synthesis of fatty acids by acetyl CoA carboxylase and fatty acid synthase requires a supply of cytoplasmic acetyl units (as acetyl CoA) and reducing power (as NADPH). When fatty acids are synthesized from glucose, acetyl units are formed as acetyl CoA within mitchondria by pyruvate dehydrogenase and thus there must be some means of transferring acetyl units across the mitochondrial membrane as acetyl CoA itself is not transported directly. A number of possibilities have been suggested including transport as acetate, acetylcarnitine, acetoacetate and acetyl aspartate. The following evidence, however, strongly favours citrate as the means of transferring acetyl units:—

(i) The enzymes required, citrate synthase and ATP citrate lyase, are present in adequate activity to account for observed rates of fatty acid synthesis and are present solely in the expected cell compartment, namely mitochondrial and cytoplasmic respectively. Activities of enzymes necessary for the other possible pathways appear to be on the whole insufficient.

(ii) Isolated fat cell mitochondria convert pyruvate to citrate at high rates and do not form significant amounts of other possible acetyl transferring intermediates. The mitochondria contain high activities of a transporter which exchanges citrate for malate.

(iii) ATP-citrate lyase activity extracted from adipose tissue alters with hormonal and nutritional status of the rats (see Section 3.3.3) and these alterations parallel changes in the capacity of the tissue for fatty acid synthesis. This enzyme is only found in tissues capable of fatty acid synthesis.

Continuous transfer of acetyl units as citrate requires the regeneration of mitochondrial oxaloacetate from the oxaloacetate formed in the cytoplasm by ATP-citrate lyase. This is most likely accomplished at least in rat adipose tissue by conversion of the oxaloacetate to pyruvate via cytoplasmic NAD$^+$-dependent malate dehydrogenase and the NADP$^+$-linked malic enzyme and then entry of pyruvate into mitochondria and generation of oxaloacetate by pyruvate carboxylase, an exclusively mitochondrial enzyme. In one turn of the complete 'pyruvate-citrate-malate' cycle (see Fig. 3.6), one acetyl unit is transported out of the mitochondrial compartment and reducing power is transferred from one molecule of cytoplasmic NADH to NADP$^+$. This transfer could account for much of the reducing power generated by glycolysis and form sufficient NADPH to satisfy approximately half that required by fatty acid synthesis. This fits in nicely with the calculated rate of the pentose cycle which is sufficient to supply only 50—60% of the reducing power required for fatty acid synthesis. Further evidence for the 'pyruvate-citrate-malate' cycle comes from the finding of sufficient activities of the enzymes in appropriate cell compartments and observations that the activity of malic enzyme and to some extent that of pyruvate carboxylase vary in parallel with the capacity for fatty acid synthesis (cf. ATP-citrate lyase). There is no really convincing isotopic evidence that the cycle operates but the incorporation into fatty acids of $[^{14}C]$ from $[2,3-^{14}C]$ succinate, but not $[1,4-^{14}C]$ succinate, is consistent with the pathway.

Overall, the reducing power formed by glycolysis and the pentose cycle in the cytoplasm closely matches that used by fatty acid synthesis together with glycerol phosphate and lactate formation and thus little if any reducing power can be transferred into mitochondria. As the transfer of citrate out of mitochondria is probably in exchange for malate, a short circuit of the citrate-malate-pyruvate cycle might be expected (shown in dotted arrows in Fig. 3.6). This short-circuit would necessarily involve transfer of reducing power into mitochondria and presumably therefore does not occur to any extent. It follows there must be some restriction on malate metabolism in fat cell mitochondria and that malate entering in exchange for citrate must subsequently leave on the separate dicarboxylate transporter. The rate of fatty acid synthesis from glucose does not appear ever to be limited by the supply of NADPH but mechanisms must be present which ensure that an appropriate proportion comes from malic enzyme and from the pentose cycle.

3.3.3 Long-term regulation of fatty acid synthesis

Adipose tissue from starved animals has a greatly diminished capacity for converting glucose to fatty acids and contains much reduced activities of a number of enzymes involved in fatty acid synthesis (Fig. 3.7). These enzymes include not only those directly involved in the pathway but also those involved in the provision of reducing power. On refeeding there are parallel increases in both fatty acid synthesis from glucose and the enzyme activities and indeed these attain levels greater than those of the controls. Very similar changes to starvation are seen with

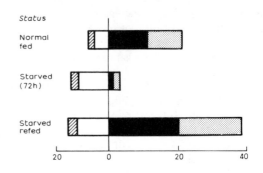

Fig. 3.7 Effects of starvation and re-feeding on glucose metabolism in rat epididymal adipose tissue. Total length of the bars represents total glucose uptake of pads incubated *in vitro* in the presence of insulin with the sections representing incorporation into glyceride glycerol ▨, lactate plus pyruvate ☐, fatty acid ■ and CO_2 ▨. Data of [9]. Activities of many enzymes are reduced following 72h starvation and greatly increase on re-feeding including in:— *Glycolysis*: hexokinase; *pathways of NADPH production*: glucose 6-phosphate dehydrogenase, 6-phosphogluconate dehydrogenase, malic enzyme; *fatty acid synthesis*: ATP-citrate lyase, acetyl CoA carboxylase, fatty acid synthase.

alloxan-diabetes and these are reversed by insulin treatment. The changes in enzyme activity are presumed to be the result of specific repression or induction of the enzymes concerned. Unequivocal evidence for this requires the use of specific antibodies so that the turnover rate of the enzymes can be calculated (see Section 2.5.3) and this has not yet been accomplished in most cases. Nevertheless, it appears that much of the pathway from glucose to fatty acids is under long term control and that the changes seen for example in starvation or diabetes are important in the large diminution in fatty acid synthesis capacity. Changes in the plasma concentration of hormones, and more particularly in insulin, are assumed to be important in initiating the

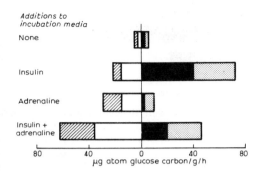

Fig. 3.8 Effects of insulin and adrenaline on glucose metabolism in rat epididymal adipose tissue. Histograms show glucose metabolism to glyceride glycerol ▨, lactate plus pyruvate ☐, fatty acids ■ and CO_2 ▨ by pads incubated *in vitro* in the presence of the hormones indicated. Data of [10].

changes in specific enzyme synthesis but direct evidence is lacking. This is partly because convincing changes in activity are not consistently obtained with *in vitro* preparations even after long periods of exposure to insulin or other hormones.

Laboratory rats are usually fed a diet containing less than 5% by weight lipid. If the proportion is increased to 30–40% the capacity of adipose tissue to convert glucose to fatty acids is almost entirely lost; after 2 or 3 weeks on the diet even the amount of pyruvate dehydrogenase in the tissue is diminished. The mechanisms involves in these changes are not clear; only a small reduction in circulating insulin is seen. Samples of human adipose tissue synthesize little or no fatty acid from glucose. These samples have invariably been taken from Western subjects and it is possible that the lack of fatty acid synthesis is related to their high fat diet.

3.3.4 Acute regulation of fatty acid synthesis
Very striking changes in glucose metabolism are observed following brief exposure of adipose tissue to insulin or adrenaline (Fig. 3.8). Both insulin and adrenaline stimulate overall glucose uptake by the tissue. This undoubtedly involves acceleration of glucose transport but the mechanisms are entirely obscure. The metabolism of glucose within the tissue is very different in the presence of insulin from that in the presence of adrenaline. It can be seen (Fig. 3.8) that insulin stimulates conversion of glucose to all end products but especially to fatty acids whereas adrenaline only stimulates conversion to lactate plus pyruvate and glyceride glycerol and, indeed, in the presence of insulin may actually inhibit fatty acid synthesis. These observations indicate that insulin causes activation of the pathway segment [pyruvate → fatty acids] while adrenaline does not and may even inhibit flux through this segment. Recent studies indicate that these effects may be brought about largely by parallel alteration of the activities of pyruvate dehydrogenase and acetyl CoA carboxylase (Fig. 3.9). Both enzymes have interconvertible active and inactive forms. How interaction of insulin and adrenaline with receptors on the outside of the cell membrane can lead to acute changes in the activity of both a cytoplasmic and a mitochondrial enzyme system is an intriguing problem, particularly since cyclic $3'5'$ AMP and cyclic $3'5'$ AMP-sensitive protein kinase do not appear to have any direct effects on either system. An understanding of the mechanisms involved should not only add to our knowledge of the regulation of fatty acid synthesis in general terms but may offer a clue to the mechanism of action of insulin. As pointed out above, no really satisfactory explanation exists of this hormone's action on a number of other intracellular processes including glycogen synthesis and lipolysis.

The pyruvate dehydrogenase complex in adipose tissue has properties similar to those of the heart complex summarized in Fig. 3.5. Brief exposure to insulin increases the proportion in the non-phosphorylated form from about 35 to 70% of the total complex. Little change is seen on exposure to both insulin and adrenaline

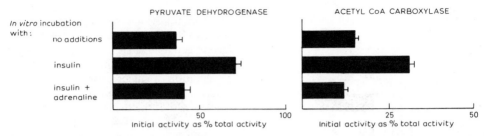

Fig. 3.9 Effects of insulin and adrenaline on the activity of pyruvate dehydrogenase and acetyl CoA carboxylase in rat epididymal fat pads. Results for pyruvate dehydrogenase initial activity are expressed as a percentage of the total activity observed after incubation of tissue extract with pyruvate dehydrogenase phosphatase in the presence of Mg^{2+} and Ca^{2+} [11]; those for acetyl CoA carboxylase initial activity are expressed at a percentage of the total activity observed after incubation of the tissue extract with citrate [12].

(Fig. 3.9). The effect of insulin could be brought about by an activation of the phosphatase or by inhibition of the kinase or both. On the basis of the complex regulatory properties of both the kinase and phosphatase a large number of possible mechanisms could be suggested. We are therefore faced again with the usual problem that discrimination between these possible mechanisms requires knowledge of changes of the intramitochondrial concentrations of the various effectors and this cannot be obtained by direct techniques on whole cell preparations. However, the effect of insulin persists during preparation of mitochondria from fat pads and is still evident after 10–20 min incubation of fat pad mitochondria with respiratory substrates other than pyruvate [13]. This rather surprising phenomenon offers some real hope that the mechanism involved in the action of insulin will be eventually ascertained. To date, it is clear that changes in the mitochondrial content of pyruvate and ATP are unlikely to be involved since in the isolated mitochondrion effects of insulin persist in the absence of pyruvate and when the ATP concentration is unaltered. It has been suggested that insulin may act through increasing the concentration of Ca^{2+} in mitochondria; Ca^{2+} is both an inhibitor of the kinase and an activator of the phosphatase. However, no direct evidence for an effect of insulin on the calcium content of mitochondria has been obtained and it appears likely that the concentration of Ca^{2+} in mitochondria is greater than the range (10^{-7} to 10^{-5} M) over which the phosphatase and kinase are sensitive to changes in Ca^{2+} concentration.

Acetyl CoA carboxylase purified from mammalian sources is active only when 10–20 protomers aggregate into long filamentous polymers of molecular weight 4 to 8 x 10^6. Aggregation is favoured in the presence of citrate whilst fatty acyl CoA or carboxylation of the enzyme by ATP Mg^{2-} in the presence of HCO_3^- favours dissociation. In fact the enzyme appears to be uniquely sensitive to fatty acyl CoA; effects are seen at concentrations below 1 μM and are reversible. The activity of acetyl CoA carboxylase is increased two-fold in extracts of insulin-treated tissue (Fig. 3.9). Insulin does not alter the total amount of the enzyme, since preincubation of extracts with citrate before assay leads to activation of the enzyme and loss of the effect of insulin. Insulin thus appears to cause an increase in the ratio of polymeric to protomeric forms and this can be demonstrated more directly using high speed centrifugation to separate the two forms. The presence of adrenaline reverses the changes seen with insulin.

Evidence has been presented that acetyl CoA carboxylase from liver may be regulated by a phosphorylation-dephosphorylation cycle [14] but no convincing evidence has been obtained that the changes observed in the adipose tissue enzyme are associated with such a cycle. Rather, it appears more likely that changes in either the concentration of citrate or fatty acyl CoA are important. One cannot eliminate completely the possibility that citrate may regulate the enzyme because of compartmentation of the metabolite between mitochondria and cytoplasm but the complete lack of any correlation between tissue concentrations of citrate and the initial activity of acetyl CoA carboxylase in extracts does suggest that regulation by citrate may not be of physiological importance. Perhaps most striking is the observed eightfold rise in citrate concentration on incubation of adipose tissue in the presence of pyruvate without any appreciable increase in the activity of acetyl CoA carboxylase [12]. On the other hand, there is some evidence for an inverse correlation between whole tissue fatty acyl CoA levels and the initial activity of acetyl CoA carboxylase in tissues incubated with insulin, suggesting that acute regulation may be through changes in the cytoplasmic concentration of fatty acyl CoA. The concentration of fatty acyl CoA in fat cells calculated on the basis of this metabolite being evenly distributed throughout the cell is, however, about 100—150 μM (calculation in other tissues would give similar values). This is 2 or 3 orders of magnitude greater than the apparent K_i of acetyl CoA carboxylase for palmitoyl CoA; this concentration would be such as to denature most enzymes irreversibly. It must be concluded that extensive binding of fatty acyl CoA must occur within cells and this is in accord with the apparent coexistence of fatty acyl CoA with high activities of fatty acyl CoA hydrolyase within cells of many tissues. Fatty acyl CoA is known to bind strongly to membranes and many proteins; both phospholipid micelles and albumin bind palmitoyl CoA sufficiently strongly to reverse its inhibitory effects on acetyl CoA carboxylase activity. One strong possibility is that

fatty acyl CoA is bound very largely to a specific 'carrier protein' and a likely candidate is a small protein (mol. wt. 12 000) known as 'Z protein' or 'fatty acid binding protein' [15, 16]. Whatever the sites to which fatty acyl CoA is bound, it is clear that if binding to these sites is regulated, then measurements of the whole tissue concentration of this metabolite will not necessarily reflect changes in its free cytoplasmic concentration and are thus of rather doubtful value.

The parallel changes in the activity of pyruvate dehydrogenase with those of acetyl CoA carboxylase suggest that the hormonal regulation of these enzymes may be closely linked. For example, changes in cytoplasmic concentration of fatty acyl CoA might initiate changes in the activity of both enzymes if cytoplasmic levels of fatty acyl CoA can regulate the mitochondrial concentration of an effector of the pyruvate dehydrogenase system. Fatty acyl CoA may be a physiological inhibitor of the mitochondrial transport of adenine nucleotides and it has been argued that a decrease in the cytoplasmic concentration of fatty acyl CoA may lead to a decrease in the mitochondrial ATP/ADP ratio and thus activation of pyruvate dehydrogenase [17]. However, the persistence of the effect of insulin during isolation and subsequent incubation of mitochondria from fat pads would appear to rule out this possibility [13].

3.3.5 Regulation of esterification of fatty acids

Very little is known about the regulation of this pathway. The enzymes involved are difficult to study because of the tendency of the lipid substrates and products to bind to proteins or form miscelles. Glycerol phosphate in adipose tissue is largely derived from glucose since the tissue contains little glycerokinase activity. At first sight, it might seem likely that the concentration of glycerol phosphate should be important in the regulation of esterification because then it might be argued that triglyceride synthesis would be stimulated when glucose availability was high. However, the cytoplasmic NAD⁺-glycerol phosphate dehydrogenase appears to catalyse a step close to equilibrium and the concentration of glycerol phosphate appears to be determined by the cytoplasmic dihydroxyacetone phosphate concentration and the $NADH/NAD^+$ ratio (Fig. 3.9). Neither of these parameters necessarily change in parallel with glucose availability or the rate of glycolysis. In fact, there is very little correlation between the whole tissue concentration of glycerol phosphate and the rate of esterification. It would seem likely that either the concentration of fatty acyl CoA is all important or that one or more of the enzymes involved in triglyceride synthesis is subject to other (as yet unrecognized) forms of regulation. The lack of knowledge concerning the disposition of fatty acyl CoA in cells clearly limits progress in this field and in particular our understanding of the relationship between the free concentration of this metabolite and the rate of its esterification (Fig. 3.10).

3.4 Carbohydrate synthesis in liver

3.4.1 General aspects of liver metabolism
The liver may be regarded as the central metabolic 'homeostat' in the body. Thus, it responds to the very variable quantity and quality of nutrients in the incoming portal blood by performing the appropriate metabolic interconversions so that the composition of the blood leaving by the hepatic vein remains relatively constant and independent of the external environment.

It is not surprising, therefore, to find that the liver is capable of performing most of the reactions involved in the synthesis, degradation and possible interconversions of carbohydrate, fats and amino acids. It is indeed the only organ with the capacity to produce urea, ketone bodies and lipoprotein, and is the major site for the synthesis of purines, steroids and glucose.

3.4.2 The importance of gluconeogenesis
Gluconeogenesis may superficially appear to be a pathway of limited significance in man in the 'developed' areas of the world. Whilst, however, it is true that glucose synthesis is low in the well-fed state, it still plays an important role in overall metabolism (Fig. 3.11). Quantitatively the major substrates for gluconeogenesis are lactate and alanine (end-products of muscle metabolism) with glycerol (derived from triglyceride in adipose tissue and liver itself) a poor third. Glutamine is also glucogenic, but it seems likely that the kidney may be more active in this respect than the liver. Other amino acids (e.g. histidine, proline) may contribute to glucose synthesis, but probably to a small extent only *in vivo* (Fig. 3.11).

Animals are unable to effect a net synthesis of carbohydrate from fatty acids; there is no glyoxalate cycle. [¹⁴C]Acetate may give rise to [¹⁴C]glucose but this is a result of the redistribution of [¹⁴C] in intermediates during citrate cycle activity; it does not indicate *net* synthesis. The one exception is propionate which is a good precursor of glucose in many species. It is particularly important in ruminants where carbohydrate is derived almost totally from propionate plus lactate (indicated by the daily production of up to 2 kg of lactose by the lactating cow).

When dietary glucose is low, as in starvation or the newborn in monogastric mammals or as usual in ruminants, blood glucose levels are maintained exclusively by increased gluconeogenesis. In the diabetic state, the elevated blood glucose arises from a combination of impaired peripheral glucose uptake and increased hepatic gluconeogenesis.

3.4.3 The pathway of gluconeogenesis
Gluconeogenesis has many reactions in common with glycolysis. There are three points at which the pathways differ — the interconversions of glucose and glucose 6-phosphate, fructose

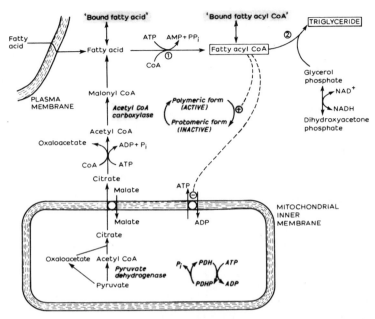

Fig. 3.10 Metabolic role of fatty acyl CoA in adipose tissue. The enzymes involved in the formation of fatty acyl CoA from fatty acids, fatty acyl CoA synthetase (1) and the esterification of fatty acyl CoA (2) are microsomal and so are the systems (not shown) for interconverting saturated and unsaturated fatty acyl CoA.

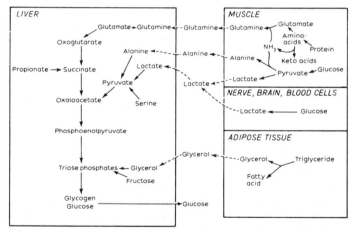

Fig. 3.11 Sources of the major substrates for gluconeogenesis in liver and their entry into the pathway. In resting man starved for 24h the daily rate of gluconeogenesis is about 150g of which some 30% is derived from lactate (+ pyruvate), 10% from glycerol and the remainder from amino acids. After 5-6 weeks of starvation the rate declines to about 80g per day of which 60% comes from lactate (+ pyruvate) and 20% each from glycerol and amino acids.

6-phosphate and fructose 1, 6-diphosphate, and phosphoenolpyruvate and pyruvate (Fig. 3.12).

The precise pathway from pyruvate to phosphoenolpyruvate is dependent both on species and the substrate involved. In the rat, phosphoenolpyruvate carboxykinase (PEPCK) is almost totally cytoplasmic. Since oxaloacetate does not cross the inner mitochondrial membrane, its transport depends upon its conversion to either aspartate or malate (see 1.3.2). Both of these cross the membrane and regenerate oxaloacetate in the cytoplasm. When cytoplasmic NADH is available for gluconeogenesis, e.g. when lactate is the substrate, oxaloacetate leaves the mitochondrion as aspartate. Conversely, where cytoplasmic NADH is low (e.g. pyruvate, propionate as substrates), malate is the intermediate (Fig. 3.12). In other species, phosphoenolpyruvate carboxykinase activity is typically found in both the cytoplasmic and mitochondrial compartments (Table 3.1). Where the enzyme is mitochondrial, phosphoenolpyruvate may cross the inner membrane in exchange for citrate (see 1.3.2).

The mitochondrial and cytoplasmic phosphoenolpyruvate carboxykinases are immunologically distinct. In addition, the increase in total phosphoenolpyruvate carboxykinase activity in livers from starved animals is mainly attributable to changes in the amount of the cytoplasmic enzyme; the mitochondrial activity does not respond to nutritional or hormonal stimuli. In all probability, both enzymic activities are important for gluconeogenesis in the intact animal. How the relative activities *in vivo* vary from one state to another remains to be resolved.

Gluconeogenesis from alanine occurs by yet another metabolic route. Oxaloacetate leaves the mitochondrion as aspartate which releases its nitrogen through the urea cycle and thereby gives rise to malate. This in turn regenerates oxaloacetate and NADH (Fig. 3.12).

Table 3.1 Intracellular distribution of phosphoenolpyruvate carboxykinase in livers from fed animals of various species.

Species	% of total	
	Mitochondria	Cytoplasm
Rat ⎫ Mouse ⎬	5	95
Guinea pig	80	20
Man	60	40
Cow ⎫ Sheep ⎬	50	50
Rabbit ⎫ Pigeon ⎬	95	5

Table 3.2 Factors affecting gluconeogenesis in liver.

Stimulation	Inhibition
Short-term starvation	Long-term starvation
Glucagon	Insulin
Catecholamines	Alcohol
Cyclic AMP	Tryptophan
Glucocorticoids	
Exercise	
Vasopressin	
Fatty acids (some species)	

3.4.4 Factors affecting gluconeogenesis

Gluconeogenesis *in vitro* is affected by a number of treatments and agents (Table 3.2). In particular, much attention has been given experimentally to the actions of fatty acids, glucagon, the catecholamines and glucocorticoids.

High concentrations of fatty acids increase glucose production in perfused livers from starved rats. This has been attributed both to the increased production of acetyl CoA, an activator of pyruvate carboxylase, and to the raised mitochondrial $NADH/NAD^+$ ratio (a result of β-oxidation), favouring malate formation from oxaloacetate. In the guinea pig, however, similar concentrations of fatty acids

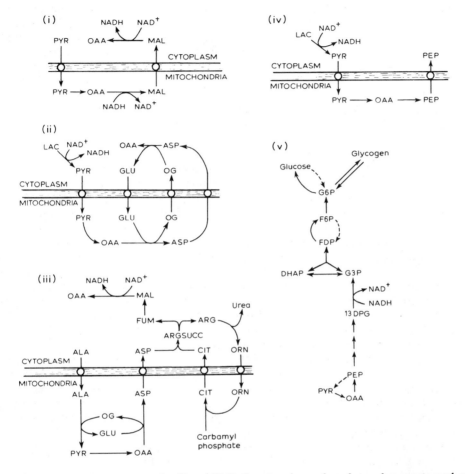

Fig. 3.12 Pathways of gluconeogenesis. (i) – (iii) Pathways where phosphoenolpyruvate carboxy-kinase (PEPCK) is cytoplasmic; (iv) where PEPCK is mitochondrial. (i) Pyruvate as substrate; (ii) lactate as substrate; (iii) alanine as substrate; (iv) lactate as substrate. (v) Common path from PEP to glucose and glycogen.

Arrows show *net* flux during gluconeogenesis. Dotted lines indicate possible 'futile cycle' reactions. ALA – alanine; ARG – arginine; ARGSUCC – argininosuccinate; ASP – aspartate; CIT – citrulline; DHAP – dihydroxyacetone phosphate; 13 DPG – 1, 3-diphosphoglycerate; FDP – fructose 1, 6-diphosphate; FUM – fumarate; F6P – fructose 6-phosphate; GLU – glutamate; G3P – glyceraldehyde 3-phosphate; G6P – glucose 6-phosphate; LAC – lactate; MAL – malate; OAA – oxaloacetate; OG – 2-oxoglutarate; ORN – ornithine; PEP – phosphoenolpyruvate; PYR – pyruvate. ◯ specific porter system in inner mitochondrial membrane; details omitted for clarity.

59

inhibit gluconeogenesis. This may be connected with the presence of a mitochondrial phosphoenolpyruvate carboxykinase; the displacement of the malate dehydrogenase equilibrium probably reduces the oxaloacetate available to the enzyme.

Fatty acids at concentrations that occur naturally do not, however, alter gluconeogenesis in the isolated liver. Equally, the evidence derived from whole animal experiments and from limited measurements in man does not show a clear relationship between fatty acids and hepatic gluconeogenesis. It therefore remains hard to assess the real significance of the activation effect *in vitro.*

Glucagon stimulates glycogenolysis, gluconeogenesis, ketogenesis and ureogenesis in the isolated perfused liver. Only the first two of these processes are, however, sensitive to the range of concentrations of the hormone normally encountered. The effect on glycogen breakdown is clearly explicable in terms of the increased intracellular cyclic AMP concentration; this leads to activation of phosphorylase kinase and hence of phosphorylase activity. The effect on gluconeogenesis is less easily understood. Measurements of metabolites in livers perfused with glucagon and either lactate or glutamine indicate a point of action between malate-aspartate and phosphoenolpyruvate. This is consistent with phosphoenolpyruvate carboxykinase being rate-limiting, but it is difficult to be precise since the exact concentration and intracellular distributions, particularly of oxaloacetate, are far from easy to ascertain. Since similar effects may be elicited with cyclic AMP, it seems reasonable to infer that the action of glucagon is mediated through this compound.

Adrenaline also exerts effects similar to those of glucagon; the cyclic AMP concentration is again increased. The amount of adrenaline required for observable changes is, however, unphysiologically high, so that it is very unlikely that this hormone is directly important *in vivo*; its actions are more directed towards peripheral tissue metabolism. Noradrenaline may be more important, however, in that the liver in the whole animal is supplied by the splanchic (adrenergic) and vagus (cholinergic) nerves. Stimulation of the former increases glycogenolysis, and of the latter glycogen synthesis. This may well reflect an important control mechanism *in vivo.*

Glucocorticoids play a major role in the regulation of gluconeogenesis, not so much by stimulating flux directly but by permitting responses to other treatments such as starvation, diabetes and glucagon. Adrenalectomy has little if any effect on glucose synthesis in the fed rat, but blocks the increase in acute starvation, so that animals treated in this way are prone to die from hypoglycaemia. Again, glucagon is only effective in animals with normal adrenal function. Since the cyclic AMP concentration rises as expected, the effect of corticosteroid is probably on the pathway itself, rather than at the level of hormone binding or primary interactions.

A major factor regulating gluconeogenesis *in vivo* in undoubtedly substrate supply. Since the plasma concentrations of lactate, glycerol, amino acids, etc., are dependent on the interplay of many factors (including catecholamines, insulin and steroids) acting peripherally, it is clear that this is a further, less direct, way in which hormones influence gluconeogenesis.

3.4.5 Relationship of gluconeogenesis to glycolysis and glycogen metabolism

Liver plays a key role in the maintenance of blood glucose concentrations. After a meal, when the portal blood glucose concentration is high, the sugar is converted to glycogen or *via* glycolysis to fatty acid. Between meals or, more particularly, during short periods of starvation, when the supply of glucose in the blood is at a premium, glucose is both released by glycogenolysis and synthesized through gluconeogenesis. Glucose transport across the liver cell membrane appears to be very rapid and never limiting, so that the intracellular glucose concentration is similar to that in the blood. This indicates that, in the first instance at least, the regulation of glucose uptake or output by the liver depends on the relative activities of glucokinase and glucose 6-phosphatase, both of which catalyse non-equilibrium reactions. This postulate is supported by the observation that the amounts of these two enzymes are regulated inversely by varying nutritional and hormonal environments. In starvation or diabetes, for example, glucose 6-phosphatase activity increases several-fold, whilst glucokinase becomes barely detectable. It is also of interest that glucokinase has not been found in ruminants where the liver is primarily concerned with glucose production.

While these long-term mechanisms may restrict the extent of ATP hydrolysis by 'futile cycling' between the two enzymes, it is probable that some degree of such 'cycling' is a normal phenomenon. In the short term, cycling may be regulated less by the kinetic properties of the enzymes than by compartmentation arising from the association of glucose 6-phosphatase with the endoplasmic reticulum.

3.4.6 The role of phosphofructokinase and fructose 1, 6-diphosphatase

Experiments with labelled substrates have indicated that there may be again some measurable cycling at the level of fructose 6-phosphate. Such cycling may serve both as a means of heat production and also as a 'fine' control whereby flux may be rapidly altered, albeit at the expense of ATP hydrolysis.

Liver phosphofructokinase resembles the heart enzyme (see 3.2.1) in its sensitivity to activation by AMP, ADP and P_i and inhibition by ATP and citrate. Fructose 1, 6-diphosphatase is strongly inhibited by AMP. Although one might think that AMP is an obvious candidate for a regulator, there is no evidence to show that changes in flux correlate with changes in the concentration of AMP or, indeed, of those of other effectors. It may be that these modulate activity of the 'cycle', but do not ultimately determine flux.

Since neither enzyme is markedly sensitive to long-term control (by induction or repression), the nature of the regulatory mechanism at this step is still far from clear. Possibilities still to be fully explored are enzyme-enzyme interaction and phosphorylation mechanisms (see Table 1.5).

3.4.7 The role of pyruvate kinase

Liver pyruvate kinase differs from the muscle enzyme in that it exhibits sigmoid kinetics with phosphoenolpyruvate, is strongly activated by fructose 1, 6-diphosphate, and inhibited by ATP and alanine. Under gluconeogenic conditions, appreciable pyruvate kinase activity would permit yet a third 'futile cycle'. Changes in hepatic fructose 1, 6-diphosphate may well be sufficient, however, to produce activation under glycolytic, and inhibition under gluconeogenic, conditions. Fructose 1, 6-diphosphate is known, nevertheless, to bind strongly to aldolase, so that total concentrations measured may not reflect the actual amount accessible to pyruvate kinase. Yet a further possibility for a control mechanism is suggested by the observation of protein kinase-dependent phosphorylation of liver pyruvate kinase (Table 1.5).

3.4.8 The role of pyruvate carboxylase

Although pyruvate carboxylase is not exclusively a gluconeogenic enzyme, it plays an important role in controlling the formation of mitochondrial oxaloacetate from lactate, pyruvate, alanine, serine, etc. Enzyme activity is dependent on acetyl CoA and is inhibited by ADP. The increase in acetyl CoA in conditions of accelerated gluconeogenesis is consistent with a short-term control exerted through this intermediate.

3.4.9 The role of phosphoenolpyruvate carboxykinase

The hypothesis that phosphoenolpyruvate carboxykinase is rate-limiting for gluconeogenesis is supported by the following observations, (i) Phosphoenolpyruvate carboxykinase is the first enzyme of gluconeogenesis proper. Although the K'_{eq} is only 2.8, such measurements as have been made suggest that the enzyme does not catalyse an equilibrium reaction *in vivo*. (ii) The concentrations of malate and aspartate, generally assumed to be in equilibrium with oxaloacetate, are consistent with a drop in total oxaloacetate during increased gluconeogenesis. (iii) Total phosphoenolpyruvate carboxykinase protein is increased during periods of glucose synthesis, and vice versa.

Extensive searches have been conducted to identify possible effectors of phosphoenolpyruvate carboxykinase. All to no avail; none of the many metabolites tested, including cyclic AMP, has any effect at physiological concentrations. In addition, the enzyme as isolated is a monomer (mol. wt. approx. 70 000), an unusual property for a putative regulatory enzyme. Lardy has suggested that phosphoenolpyruvate carboxykinase may be activated by a Fe^{2+}-containing protein whose activity is itself subject to regulation. If one takes the view that glucagon acts through intracellular cyclic AMP, then it is not unreasonable to suspect that such a protein may be modified by a protein kinase-dependent process.

Although gluconeogenesis may be stimulated under conditions where there is no apparent change in assayable phosphoenolpyruvate carboxykinase, it is clear that, in the longer term, the increase in total enzyme protein is important for the maintenance of increased flux.

In liver, total phosphoenolpyruvate carboxykinase rises in starvation and diabetes, and, *in vitro*, in response to glucocorticoids and glucagon; it falls with insulin and at high glucose concentrations. The effect of glucagon may also be elicited with dibutyryl cyclic AMP (a less metabolizable analogue of cyclic AMP).

Immunoprecipitation studies have shown that changes in assayable enzyme activity parallel changes in total phosphoenolpyruvate carboxykinase protein. Such techniques also permit the measurement of enzyme synthesis (and degradation) during steady-state conditions when, of course, there is no observable change in *activity*. The use of actinomycin D, cordycepin (inhibitor of mRNA synthesis), and cycloheximide (an inhibitor of mRNA translation) has shown that, whilst glucocorticoid stimulation is at the transcriptional level, the effect of cyclic AMP appears to be upon some post-transcriptional process (possibly chain initiation). This has been confirmed in subsequent immunoprecipitation experiments.

In an isolated minimally-transformed liver cell line (Reuber H-35 cells), phosphoenolpyruvate carboxykinase synthesis ceases rapidly after removal of dibutyryl cyclic AMP. This is not due to increased turnover of phosphoenolpyruvate carboxykinase mRNA, since dibutyryl cyclic AMP can restore full synthesis even in the absence of *de novo* RNA synthesis. These observations are again consistent with an action of cyclic AMP at the post-transcriptional level.

Insulin decreases phosphoenolpyruvate carboxykinase synthesis in a manner similar to that consequent upon the removal of cyclic AMP. There is evidence that insulin administration causes a fall in intracellular cyclic AMP in diabetic rat liver *in vivo*.

3.4.10 Hepatic gluconeogenesis and development

At birth, the blood glucose concentration in the neonatal rat drops sharply with removal of the maternal supply. After 2h, the concentration increases once more and reaches a 'normal' value after 5—6h. The drop in blood glucose at birth results in an increase of glucagon, and a decrease of insulin, secretion. The increased glucagon/insulin ratio stimulates intra-hepatic cyclic AMP production. This has two consequences. Firstly, glycogen is immediately mobilised. Secondly, phosphoenolpyruvate carboxykinase synthesis is stimulated, and gluconeogenesis becomes, for the first time, a functional pathway. Activity increases rapidly, partly because enzyme degradation is inhibited during this phase. The combination of glycogenolysis and gluconeogenesis at this time is essential for carbohydrate homeostasis in the newborn.

References

[1] Cohen, P. (1976), *Control of enzyme activity,* Chapman and Hall, London.
[2] Pettit, F.H., Peiley, J.W. and Reed, L.J. (1975), *Biochem. biophys. Res. Commun.,* 65, 575-582.
[3] Cooper, R.H., Randle, P.J. and Denton, R.M. (1975), *Nature,* 257, 808-809.
[4] Wollenberger, A., Babskii, E.B., Krause, E.G., Genz, S., Blohm, D. and Bogdanova, E.V. (1973), *Biochem. biophys. Res. Commun.,* 55, 446-462.
[5] Brooker, G. (1975), *Adv. in Cyclic Nucleotide Res.,* 5.
[6] Bowman, R.H. (1964), *Biochem. J.,* 93, 13-15c.
[7] Randle, P.J. (1969), *Nature,* 221, 777.
[8] Whitehouse, S., Cooper, R.H. and Randle, P.J. (1974), *Biochem. J.,* 141, 761-774.
[9] Saggerson, E.D. and Greenbaum, A.L. (1970), *Biochem. J.,* 119, 193-218.
[10] Denton, R.M. and Halperin, M.L. (1968), *Biochem. J.,* 110, 27-38.
[11] Severson, D.L., Denton, R.M., Pask, H.T. and Randle, P.J. (1974), *Biochem. J.,* 140, 225-237.
[12] Halestrap, A.P. and Denton, R.M. (1974), *Biochem. J.,* 142, 365-377.
[13] Denton, R.M. *et al.* (1975), *Mol. and Cellular Biochem.,* 9, 27-53.
[14] Carlson, C.A. and Kim, K. (1974), *Archs. Biochem. Biophys.,* 164, 478-489.
[15] Mishkin, S. and Turcotte, R. (1974), *Biochem. biophys. Res. Commun.,* 47, 918-926.
[16] Ockner, R.K. and Manning, J.A. (1974), *J. Clin. Invest.,* 54, 326-338.
[17] Weiss, L., Löffler, G. and Wieland, O. (1974), *Hoppe Seyler's Z. physiol. Chem.,* 355, 363-377.

Suggestions for further reading

Heart and muscle energy metabolism
Randle, P.J. *et al.* (1966), *Rec. Prog. Hormone Res.,* 22, 1-44.
Newsholme, E.A. (1970), In *Essays in Cell Metabolism,* p. 189-223. ed. by Bartley, W., Kornberg, H. and Quayle, J. Wiley Interscience, London.
Neely, J.R. and Morgan, H.E. (1974), *Ann. Rev. Physiol.,* 36, 413-459.
Williamson, J.R., Safer, B., La Noue, K.F., Smith, C.M. and Walajtys, E. (1973), *Symposium Soc. Exp. Biol.,* 26, 241-281.

Pyruvate dehydrogenase
Reed, L.J. (1974), *Accounts of Chem. Res.,* 7, 40-46.
Wieland, O. *et al.* (1973), *Symp. Soc. Exp. Biol.* 27, 371-400.
Denton, R.M. *et al.* (1975), *Mol. and Cellular Biochem.,* 9, 27-53.

Citrate cycle
Lowenstein, J.M. (ed.) (1969), *Citric Acid Cycle: Control and Compartmentation.* Dekker, New York.
Randle, P.J., England, P.J. and Denton, R.M. (1970), *Biochem. J.,* 117, 677-695.
Neely, J.R., Denton, R.M., England, P.J. and Randle, P.J. (1972), *Biochem. J.,* 128, 147-159.

Adipose tissue and fat synthesis
Jeanrenaud, B. and Hepp, D. Eds. (1970), *Adipose tissue: regulation and metabolic functions,* Academic Press, New York.
Jungas, R.L. (1975), *Handbook Exp. Pharm.,* 32, (part 2), 371-401.
Denton, R.M. (1975), *Proc. Nutr. Soc.,* 34, 217-224.

Acetyl CoA carboxylase and fatty acid synthase
Numa, S. and Yamashita, S. (1974), *Current topics in Cell Reg.,* 8, 197-247.
Lane, M.D., Moss, J. and Polakis, S.E. (1974), *Current topics in Cell Reg.,* 8, 139-196.
Volpe, J.J. and Vagelos, P.R. (1973), *Ann. Rev. Biochem.,* 42, 21-60.
Halestrap, A.P. and Denton, R.M. (1974), *Biochem. J.,* 142, 365-377.

Liver
Lundquist, F. and Tygstrup, N. (eds) (1974), *Alfred Benzon Symposium No. 6,* Munksgaard; Copenhagen.

Gluconeogenesis
Arion, W.J., Wallin, B.K., Lange, A.J. and Ballas, L.M. (1975), *Molec. Cell. Biochem.,* 6, 75-83 (glucose 6-phosphatase).
Exton, J.H. (1972), *Metabolism,* 21, 945-990.
Hanson, R.W. and Garber, A.J. (1972), *Amer. J. Clin. Nutr.,* 25, 1010-1021.
Hanson, R.W., Garber, A.J., Reshef, L. and Ballard, F.J. (1973), *Amer. J. Clin. Nutr.,* 26, 55-63.
Hanson, R.W. and Mehlman, M.A., (eds.) (1976), *Gluconeogenesis.* John Wiley, New York and London.
Söling, H.-D. and Willms, (eds.) (1971), *Regulation of Gluconeogenesis.* Academic Press, New York and London.

Metabolic Cycling
Bloxham, D.P. (1974), *Int. J. Biochem,* 5, 429-435.

Phosphoenolpyruvate carboxykinase
Tilghman, S.M., Gunn, J.M., Fisher, L.M., Hanson, R.W., Reshef, L. and Ballard, F.J. (1975), *J. Biol. Chem.,* 250, 3322-3329.

Gluconeogenesis and Development
Hanson, R.W., Reshef, L. and Ballard, F.J. (1975), *Federation Proceedings,* 34, 166-171.

Index

DATE DUE

30 505 JOSTEN'S